THE DOCTORS BOOK
OF
Home Remedies®
FOR
STRONGER BONES

Titles in
The Doctors Book of Home Remedies
series

Colds and Flu
Stronger Bones

THE DOCTORS BOOK
OF
Home Remedies®
FOR
STRONGER BONES

Tips to stop osteoporosis and reverse the bone loss that affects every woman over 30

By the Editors of *Prevention*
Edited by Mary S. Kittel

RODALE

Prevention and *The Doctors Book of Home Remedies* are registered trademarks of Rodale Inc.

Printed in the United States of America on acid-free ∞, recycled paper ♻

Cover Designer: Christina Gaugler

Library of Congress Cataloging-in-Publication Data

> The doctors book of home remedies for stronger bones : tips to stop osteoporosis and reverse the bone loss that affects every woman over 30 / by the editors of Prevention ; edited by Mary S. Kittel.
> p.   cm.
> Includes index.
> ISBN 1–57954–209–3 paperback
> 1. Osteoporosis in women—Popular works.   I. Kittel, Mary S.
> RC931.O73 D63   2000
> 616.7'16—dc21   99–056548

Distributed to the book trade by St. Martin's Press

2   4   6   8   10   9   7   5   3   1   paperback

Visit us on the Web at www.rodaleremedies.com, or call us toll-free at (800) 848-4735.

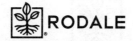

RODALE

WE **INSPIRE** AND **ENABLE** PEOPLE TO IMPROVE THEIR LIVES AND THE WORLD AROUND THEM

Notice

This book is intended as a reference volume only, not as a medical manual. The information given here is designed to help you make informed decisions about your health. It is not intended as a substitute for any treatment that may have been prescribed by your doctor. If you suspect that you have a medical problem, we urge you to seek competent medical help.

About *Prevention* Health Books

The editors of *Prevention* Health Books are dedicated to providing you with authoritative, trustworthy, and innovative advice for a healthy, active lifestyle. In all our books, our goal is to keep you thoroughly informed about the latest breakthroughs in natural healing, medical research, alternative health, herbs, nutrition, fitness, and weight loss. We cut through the confusion of today's conflicting health reports to deliver clear, concise, and definitive health information that you can trust. And we explain in practical terms what each new breakthrough means to you—so you can take immediate, practical steps to improve your health and well-being.

Every recommendation in *Prevention* Health Books is based upon interviews with highly qualified health authorities, including medical doctors and practitioners of alternative medicine. In addition, we consult with the *Prevention* Health Books Board of Advisors to ensure that all the health information is safe, practical, and up-to-date. *Prevention* Health Books are thoroughly fact-checked for accuracy, and we make every effort to verify recommendations, dosages, and cautions.

The advice in this book will help keep you well-informed about your personal choices in health care—to help you lead a happier, healthier, and longer life.

Acknowledgments

The following writers contributed to this book: Betsy Bates, Julie A. Evans, Paula Hunt, Margo Trott Mukkulainen, Elizabeth Ward

We would like to thank the following health care professionals:
James Adleberg, D.P.M., P.A.; Tammy Baker, R.D.;
Margie Bissinger, P.T.; Jacqueline Bougie, D.C.;
Margaret Burghardt, M.D.; Kitty Burroughs; Irene Catania, N.D.;
Roberto Civitelli, M.D.; Felicia Cosman, M.D.; Chad Deal, M.D.;
Michael DiMuzio, Ph.D.; Barbara Drinkwater, Ph.D.;
Diane Feskanich, Sc.D.; Trisha Lamb Feuerstein; James Fleet, Ph.D.;
Suza Francina; Theresa D. Galsworthy, R.N., O.N.C.;
Michael Gloth, M.D.; Barbara Gollman, R.D.; Allen Green, M.D.;
Robert Heaney, M.D.; Michael Holick, M.D., Ph.D.;
Michele Hooper, M.D.; Tori Hudson, N.D.; Janna Kimel;
Deborah Kipp, R.D., Ph.D.; Jane Kirby, R.D.; Bonnie Kissam;
Vasant Lad, M.A.S.C.; Joseph Lane, M.D.; Jes Bruun Lauritzen, M.D.;
Michael A. Levine, M.D.; Marjorie M. Luckey, M.D.;
Allan Magaziner, D.O.; Linda Massey, R.D., Ph.D.; Tom McCook;
Michael Moore; Scarlett Moss; Miriam Nelson, Ph.D.;
Forrest Nielson, Ph.D.; Lyn Patrick, N.D.; Colleen Pierre, R.D.;
Robert Recker, M.D.; Robert Rude, M.D.; David J. Sartoris, M.D.;
Vincent Schaller, M.D.; Mary Pullig Schatz, M.D.;
Sue A. Shapses, Ph.D.; Janet Shaw, Ph.D.; Angela Stengler, N.D.;
Mark Stengler, N.D.; Darren Streff; JoAnn (Hickey) Tall, O.M.D., L.Ac.;
Evelyn Tribole, R.D.; John Turco, M.D.; Robert Uebele, P.T.;
Bruce Watkins, Ph.D.; Connie Weaver, Ph.D.;
Densie Webb, R.D., Ph.D.; Valerie Weil, M.D.; Robert Whipple, P.T.;
Susan Whiting, Ph.D.; Russell E. Windsor, M.D.;
Leonard Wisneski, M.D.; Hillary Wright, R.D.; Tricia Yu;
Janet Zand, O.M.D., L.Ac.; Katherine Zelman, R.D.

Contents

STRONG BONES FOR LIFE 73

The power is yours. Practice smart dieting, try soothing de-stressors, and spend some time in the sun. There are simple and even pleasant steps you can take to secure a bright bone future.

LIVING WELL WITH BRITTLE BONES 95

Even if you suffer from a weak skeleton, you shouldn't have any bones about doing what you want. Read this expert advice on feeling and looking your best while guarding against injury.

ALTERNATIVE OPTIONS 113

Alternative healers who can help—who they are, what they do, and the results that you can expect.

INDEX 121

Refuse to Lose

Remember that moment as a child when you realized you were taller than one of the grown-ups in your family? Chances are, the adult with whom you could finally see eye-to-eye was Grandma.

But if you dig through your old family albums and look at your grandmother in her high school graduation photo or in her wedding gown, you're likely to see a taller and straighter-standing woman than you remember. What robbed her of inches is a condition known as degenerative bone disease, or osteoporosis. And, in a tragic number of people, osteoporosis robs more than inches. It steals independence as well. The freedom of an energetic retirement all too often is cut short by complications of broken bones caused by this gradual, insidious disease.

One out of every two women in the United States has an osteoporosis-related fracture in her lifetime, adding up to 1.5 million broken bones a year. Of them, 300,000 are hip fractures, which can lead to disability or death. One-quarter of the women over 50 who experience hip fractures die within a year. A quarter of the women who survive hip fractures require long-term care.

Another 700,000 fractures experienced annually are vertebral. Vertebral compression fractures cause not only loss of height but also deformity of the skeleton in the form of a hunchback or a stooped posture. Many vertebral fractures also lead to decades of chronic pain. Fractures of the wrist and other bones can also restrict activities and cause pain.

In the United States, 10 million people already have osteoporosis; 8 million of them are women. Another 18 million people have dangerously low bone mass, putting them at a high risk for developing the disease.

Despite its prevalence and the terrible toll it takes on the active lives of older Americans, osteoporosis is quite misunderstood. You can't depend on pain to alert you to its presence, because pain occurs very late in the disease, when fractures already have occurred. It's not like arthritis; your knees and finger joints won't ache or become stiff. The damage wrought by osteoporosis is silent, signaling its presence only when your bones begin to break.

This is a disease so underrecognized that, in a recent study of 2,314 women at risk for osteoporosis, 93 percent of the women who met the diagnosis had no idea they had it.

A Matter of Risk

Ironically, in those years when you stood on tiptoes to appear taller, your body was busy brewing the best medicine known to protect you against osteoporosis: dense, sturdy, resilient bones.

Calcium is so important to building strong bones in adolescence that our need for it increases to 1,300 milligrams a day from ages 9 to 18, up from the 800 milligrams that children need daily from ages 4 through 8.

By age 20, 98 percent of your peak bone mass should be reached, ideally providing you with enough bone to give you a comfortable safety margin for your critical postmenopausal years, when bone loss is extremely rapid. Estrogen, which is lost after menopause, also helps nurture and keep bones safe.

While genetics are a factor in your risk for osteoporosis, so are lifestyle choices. Smoking, alcohol, lack of exercise, and poor diet are part and parcel of the osteoporosis risk profile.

Here are some recognized genetic and lifestyle factors linked to greater-than-average risk of osteoporosis. Check to see how you measure up.

- Family history of osteoporosis
- History of fractures
- Caucasian or Asian race
- Childhood history of any disease that interfered with nutrition, growth, or exercise
- Slim build (women whose weight falls within the lowest quartile on weight charts)
- Amenorrhea, the abnormal cessation of menstrual periods
- Diet deficient in calcium or vitamin D
- Diet containing too much salt or caffeine
- Diets extremely deficient in protein or, ironically, diets with excess protein
- Heavy alcohol use
- Smoking
- Lack of exercise and physical activity or, inversely, excessive exercise, especially coupled with insufficient nutrition
- Estrogen deficiency (irregular menstrual history, removal of ovaries, menopause)
- Eating disorders or a history of "yo-yo" dieting
- Thyroid disease, hypercalciurea (too much excreted calcium), and certain other diseases
- Medications such as corticosteroids, anticonvulsants, barbiturates, and blood thinners

The Inside Story

Even people who fit into no specific risk category still can have osteoporosis and suffer fractures. One out of every 10 African-American women over 50 has the disease. Young women—and even men—can get it.

So whether your risks for osteoporosis are high or not, finding out how strong your bones are is always a good idea. After all, osteoporosis is a preventable disease.

Bone mass measurements, also called bone mineral density tests, can determine whether you're experiencing bone loss, and at what stage. The testing is quick, noninvasive, and doesn't hurt. There are several different methods, some more revealing than others, according to David J. Sartoris, M.D., professor of radiology and director of bone densitometry at the University of California, San Diego, School of Medicine.

A standard x-ray, for instance, doesn't show evidence of osteoporosis until 30 to 40 percent of your bone mass is gone. Scans such as ultrasounds and single x-ray absorptiometries give you a snapshot of how the bone is faring in a particular part of the body, say, in the forearm or the heel.

Since the skeleton doesn't lose bone mass uniformly, says Dr. Sartoris, the only way you can truly assess early bone loss is to get a DEXA (dual-energy x-ray absorptiometry) scan. This test looks at bone density where it matters the most—in your hips and spine.

Whereas experts once waited to look closely at bone until a woman was in menopause, Dr. Sartoris believes that approach wastes 20 years or more of potential intervention. If you're a woman between the ages of 21 and 35 and are at high risk, he recommends that you ask your doctor to order a DEXA scan. Some insurance companies might not pay for this test until you're older, but Dr. Sartoris puts the $150 cost into perspective: "Women spend that much on a dress or a pair of shoes. This is a test that could mean the difference in their futures!"

Your doctor should routinely order bone mineral density tests once you reach menopause. If you're undergoing osteoporosis treatment, you should get tested yearly.

Any time that you experience persistent back pain that doesn't go away, it could indicate a possible vertebral fracture caused by osteoporosis, and you should get an evaluation.

Where to Begin

Osteoporosis doesn't have to happen to you. It *is* preventable. By buying this book, you've already taken a major step in preventing the disease. If you already have bone loss or have already been diagnosed with the disease, the tips in this book can help maximize the treatment outlined by your doctor.

According to Dr. Sartoris, it's never too late to make the most of your bone mass, even if you have genetics and past habits working against you. If you can add even 5 percent to your peak bone mass through lifestyle changes (or medication), you'll be able to reduce your fracture risk by a whopping 40 percent.

Optimum Nutrition on page 7 introduces you to the role of nutrients, which play an undisputed part in building bone health. Calcium, phosphate, and other trace minerals form the crystalline latticework structure that gives bone its density. Vitamin D is needed for the bones to actually absorb the calcium.

The close weave of tissue that holds the calcium in the bone's matrix requires vitamins and protein to do its work. Vitamins and minerals also support hormone levels that are important to bone strength. Optimum Nutrition offers tasteful ideas for working the bone-essential nutrients into your diet.

Skeletal Strength through Exercise on page 39 offers a variety of exercises that will be part of your bone-building plan. You'll also read about methods to motivate you to move.

Keeping your bones healthy through exercise is a vital, ongoing process. But even if you've never exercised, experts say it's never too late to reap the bone-building benefits. In a Finnish study, women age 80 and above who did strength and balance training reduced their risk of falling by more than 30 percent.

Strong Bones for Life on page 73 offers you novel tips on lowering many controllable risk factors, such as smoking or excess salt, protein, or caffeine. You'll also discover count-less ways to make your lifestyle a little more bone-healthy and to protect whatever bone mass you have.

Living Well with Brittle Bones on page 95 is for the woman who refuses to compromise her quality of life and sense of adventure, despite the fact that she has osteo-porosis. Read on for travel advice, fashion tips, and many other ideas to avoid possible fractures and pain while con-tinuing to engage in your favorite activities.

Finally, Alternative Options on page 113 directs you to alternative health practitioners who have special strategies to avoid or cope with osteoporosis. Seek them out for your particular problems and concerns as a great adjunct to your doctor's care, or for an alternative approach to osteoporosis prevention and treatment.

Optimum Nutrition

"Most people think bone is a chunk of concrete, and that once it's formed, it's just there. But bone health requires the work of many nutrients to continue the remodeling process that goes on throughout life."

—Forrest H. Nielsen, Ph.D.,
center director and research nutritionist, United States Department of Agriculture Grand Forks Human Nutrition Research Center, Grand Forks, North Dakota

RICHEN YOUR FOOD AND ENRICH YOUR BONES

Adding evaporated milk to some of your favorite dishes will bring them to creamier levels of delight, while also doubling your calcium intake.

Maybe you purchase evaporated milk a few times a year to make that special sauce or dessert. But condensed milk should take a more prominent place in your cooking, according to Colleen Pierre, R.D. Try to work it into everyday cuisine, because it tastes great and also bolsters bones.

A cup of evaporated milk is loaded with 741 milligrams of calcium, versus 302 milligrams in regular fat-free (skim) milk.

What makes it so calcium-mighty? Removing more than half the water from milk causes the mineral's concentration to climb. Levels of vitamin D double, too, helping to promote calcium's uptake after digestion, not to mention improved absorption by your bones.

Pierre recommends you employ evaporated milk to:

- Mash potatoes
- Lighten coffee and tea
- Prepare condensed soups, such as tomato
- Make macaroni and cheese from a mix
- Prepare pudding and custard mixes

—Colleen Pierre, R.D., *is a nutrition consultant in Baltimore and author of* Calcium in Your Life.

CHOOSE SMART SNACKS

It's tough to get all the bone-boosting nutrition you need when you live life on the go. Have some high-nutrient stashes handy for when you can't sit down to a meal.

Snacking has a bad reputation. Supposedly, snacks wreck your appetite for better meals and promote weight gain. But often a hectic lifestyle necessitates on-the-go munching. There are times when you wouldn't have a day of well-rounded nutrition if you didn't eat in the car or at your desk.

"If you make wise choices, snacks can supply the nutrients you need for strong bones," says Hillary M. Wright, R.D.

Take figs. Four dried figs supply about 100 milligrams of calcium for only 200 or so calories. That's the same number of calories in four creme-filled sandwich cookies, without the calcium (not to mention figs' whopping 9 grams of fiber).

Wright says soy nuts—whole soybeans that have been soaked in water, then baked—are also superior snacks. Soy nuts supply isoflavones, plant substances that may boost bone density.

Tote small packages of raisins, craisins (dried cranberries), banana chips, and other dried fruits to boost your potassium and magnesium count, which are important for strong bones. Yogurt or cottage cheese also makes for a calcium-boosting pick-me-up.

—Hillary M. Wright, R.D., *is a nutritionist at Harvard Vanguard Medical Associates in Boston.*

Make the Most of Cottage Cheese

Cottage cheese is easy to dismiss, largely because of its bland appearance and flavor. But its image belies its stellar nutritional profile—not to mention its culinary potential.

Cottage cheese usually makes its appearance on restaurant diet plates, alongside fruit and lettuce. But don't shortchange cottage cheese by thinking that reducing is all it's good for.

According to Tammy T. Baker, R.D., cottage cheese packs a certain protein that, in the right amount, protects bones from thinning—*and* promotes healing, should fracture occur. So even though cottage cheese contains about half the calcium of milk and yogurt, it's still a contender when it comes to bone health.

And yes, cottage cheese is available in a variety of fat levels, so you can still reap its benefits with virtually little or no fat and cholesterol.

Baker offers the following ways to recast cottage cheese with some twenty-first-century pizzazz.

• Blend 2 cups of cottage cheese with 1 cup of thick and chunky salsa, or with a 1-ounce packet of dry salad dressing mix. Use this as a dip or as a topping for baked potatoes.

• Top a bagel with cottage cheese and fruit instead of cream cheese.

• Stir cottage cheese into warm or cold pasta dishes or salads.

• Blend cottage cheese with milk, sugar, and vanilla extract to use as a topping for French toast or pancakes. Or layer this mixture with your favorite cold cereal and fruit for a breakfast parfait or snack.

—Tammy T. Baker, R.D., *is spokesperson for the American Dietetic Association in Cave Creek, Arizona.*

DRINK YOUR CALCIUM

Calcium comes in more beverages than the one that puts a white mustache on your upper lip.

If you have allergies to or avoid cow's milk, fortified juices are another way to get calcium, says Barbara Gollman, R.D. But some juices are more calcium-friendly than others.

Look for those containing calcium citrate malate, a form of supplemental calcium considered superior because it's the one most absorbable by the body. You can find this form in juice brands such as Tropicana, Gerber, and Beechnut.

Health food stores and some supermarkets stock soy and rice milks fortified with calcium and vitamin D. Try these nondairy drinks in place of milk for breakfast cereal, whitening coffee, or just straight up. Like their cow's milk cousin, rice milk and soy milk are even available in chocolate and strawberry flavors.

Here's a smooth and refreshing way to drink your calcium.

Nondairy Smoothie

1 cup frozen fruit, such as berries and banana
   chunks

½ cup calcium-added orange juice
½ cup cold fortified soy milk

Whip all ingredients in a blender, and enjoy the calcium equivalent of one glass of whole milk.

—Barbara Gollman, R.D., *is spokesperson for the American Dietetic Association in Dallas and author of* The Phytopia Cookbook.

GET YOUR DAIRY—DISCOMFORT-FREE

Dairy doesn't agree with you? Don't ditch it altogether. You might be able to tolerate more calcium-rich milk products than you think.

If you're lactose intolerant, no one has to tell you that bloating, gas, and diarrhea are the unpleasant side effects of dairy foods.

But dairy foods affect everyone differently, so you need to find your lactose limit, advises Tammy T. Baker, R.D. Fortunately, lactose intolerance might not mean your last spoonful of your favorite yogurt.

She offers hope for dismayed dairy lovers with these tips.

• Drink milk with food. Milk is one of the most lactose-laden dairy foods, but downing it with food helps minimize any ill effects by slowing lactose digestion.

• Lean toward aged, hard cheeses. American, Cheddar, Swiss, Colby, and Parmesan are low-lactose choices.

- Feed on fat, in moderation. Higher-fat dairy foods, such as 2% reduced-fat milk and most regular cheeses, seem to mitigate lactose troubles.
- Focus on the fermented. Yogurt and buttermilk contain cultures that break down some of the lactose for you.
- When dining out, bring along a dairy digestive product in pill or liquid form, which provides the lactase enzyme your body lacks.

—**Tammy T. Baker, R.D.,** *is spokesperson for the American Dietetic Association in Cave Creek, Arizona.*

Reap Calcium from Your Greens

Dairy products don't have the only corner on calcium. Vegetables contain calcium, too, but you have to be resourceful in order to make produce a major calcium source.

There's no doubt that green, leafy vegetables are valuable calcium sources, particularly broccoli, bok choy, turnip greens, and kale. But there's good and bad news about the calcium that plants can provide.

First, the good news. Generally speaking, calcium from vegetables is just as available to the body as the calcium in milk, according to calcium expert Connie M. Weaver, Ph.D. One surprising exception: spinach. Nearly all of its calcium goes right through you, bound up by plant substances known as oxalates.

What's the downside? The question of quantity, she says. While the body can absorb the calcium contained in most green, leafy vegetables, there just isn't a lot for the taking. For example, you must eat more than 2½ cups of cooked broccoli or almost 2 cups of kale to get the calcium of 8 ounces of milk.

In other words, if you're going to try to make vegetables your main calcium source, you'd better like gigantic salads and be willing to find ways to work greens into most of your dishes.

This dish packs 489 grams of calcium by combining an entire pound of broccoli with dairy products.

Broccoli with Lemon Sauce

1   pound broccoli florets
1   cup fresh parsley
½   teaspoon onion powder
2   tablespoons ricotta cheese
½   cup low-fat buttermilk
    Sprinkling of dried tarragon
    Juice of half a lemon
    Pepper, to taste

Steam the broccoli until tender, about 8 minutes.

Meanwhile, in a food processor, finely chop the parsley with the onion powder and ricotta.

With the motor running, pour in the buttermilk, tarragon, and lemon juice. Process just until combined.

Drizzle the sauce over the broccoli and lightly sprinkle pepper on top.

Serves 2 to 4.

—Connie M. Weaver, Ph.D., *is a professor and head of the department of foods and nutrition at Purdue University in West Lafayette, Indiana.*

BE INVENTIVE WITH POWDERED MILK

You don't have to drink it straight to get powdered milk's impressive nutritional benefits.

A tablespoon of nonfat dry milk powder contains 94 milligrams of calcium. That's a third of the calcium contained in 8 ounces of fat-free milk—all for a mere 27 calories!

You can hardly find fault with that, except that powdered milk, when mixed with water, has the consistency (and some say the taste) of flour and water. So think of what you can sneak it in with, suggests Colleen Pierre, R.D.

Pierre promotes stirring a tablespoon of powdered milk into hot cereals prepared with water (like oatmeal or cream of wheat). She also suggests mixing it into hot cocoa or condensed cream soups. You can thicken casseroles with powdered dry milk. And here's the best tip—if you want to appeal to your and your children's sweet tooth, stir a tablespoon or two into homemade dough to pump up the calcium count of cookies.

Nobody will notice, but your skeleton will.

—Colleen Pierre, R.D., *is a nutrition consultant in Baltimore and author of* Calcium in Your Life.

CHOOSE YOUR CALCIUM CAREFULLY

Store shelves stock a dizzying array of calcium supplements. Arm yourself with these few simple facts for the best selection.

You can chew them, drink them in hot water, or swallow them whole. Some look and taste like chocolate candy. Some seem large enough to choke a goat. You know you need more calcium, so how do you choose?

First off, focus on form. According to Susan J. Whiting, Ph.D., calcium carbonate is your best bet. True, the calcium citrate form may be absorbed slightly better by the body. But it costs more, and over the years the dollars add up. Calcium carbonate is still a good supplement, without making you broke, she adds.

You'll need to splurge for calcium citrate, however, if you suffer from atrophic gastritis, or low stomach acid. People with this condition can absorb calcium only in citrate form.

Also, question quality. Dr. Whiting recommends supplements sporting the USP insignia. USP stands for United States Pharmacopeia, an independent group that sets pharmaceutical standards. The USP stamp of approval means your calcium supplement will dissolve properly in your body, allowing absorption.

Finally, consider vitamin D. If you're not drinking enough vitamin D–fortified milk, or if you don't regularly take a multivitamin with D, you're probably falling short of this nutrient, which is needed to enhance the absorption of calcium in the body. Take a calcium supplement that will give you 400 to 600 international units (IU) of vitamin D and 1,500 milligrams of calcium daily, advises Dr. Whiting.

> **—Susan J. Whiting, Ph.D.,** *is an assistant dean and professor in the college of pharmacy and nutrition at the University of Saskatchewan in Saskatoon, Canada.*

TAKE CALCIUM WITH FOOD

When's the best time to take vitamin and mineral supplements? Probably your favorite time of the day—mealtime.

It's not enough just to take your calcium tablet every day. The frequency and time that you take it count.

Your best bet is to take calcium with meals, advises Susan J. Whiting, Ph.D. Although both calcium carbonate and citrate forms are quite absorbable, taking supplements with food allows peak calcium absorption. There's one exception: Avoid taking calcium with high-fiber wheat bran cereal, which can reduce absorption by 25 percent.

Meals also can serve as reminders, jogging your memory to consume calcium pills, adds Dr. Whiting. Taking supplements as part of a daily routine will keep you on track.

When it comes to amount, limit calcium to 500 milligrams per dose to promote the body's absorption. And don't combine calcium with any iron-containing supplement because calcium interferes with the body's iron uptake. That means you should buy a multivitamin that has either calcium or iron, but not both. If you need extra iron, take the two supplements at different times.

—Susan J. Whiting, Ph.D., *is an assistant dean and professor in the college of pharmacy and nutrition at the University of Saskatchewan in Saskatoon, Canada.*

CHOOSE YOUR ANTACIDS CAREFULLY

Phosphorus is second only to calcium as the most abundant mineral in the body and in bones. And you get plenty in your diet—but certain antacids could be depleting your supply.

Phosphorus is a vital part of every cell's genetic material. Strong bones depend on it. Along with calcium, phosphorus lends structure to your skeleton, according to Hillary M. Wright, R.D.

Phosphorus is found in protein-rich foods, so if you're eating right, you're getting what you need, says Wright—unless you're taking antacids.

Wright warns that chronic consumption of antacids that contain aluminum hydroxide causes phosphorus excretion from the body, resulting in bones that can weaken to the point of fracture. Switch to antacids like Tums, which is made of calcium carbonate. Chewing on Tums contributes to your daily calcium quota, while preserving phosphorus.

—Hillary M. Wright, R.D., *is a nutritionist at Harvard Vanguard Medical Associates in Boston.*

MAKE SURE TO GET PLENTY OF MAGNESIUM

Magnesium appears to influence bone health in myriad ways, many of which are not fully understood. Nevertheless, there's no question about the importance of getting enough of this mineral.

Researchers aren't exactly sure why magnesium promotes bone health, but they know that bones suffer without this magnificent mineral. So be sure to get a daily supply, says Robert K. Rude, M.D. And that's at least 320 milligrams a day, the Recommended Dietary Allowance (RDA).

Magnesium is found primarily in legumes, vegetables, and whole grains. Make a magnesium-laden meal from bulgur wheat by preparing store-bought tabbouleh salad mix according to the package directions and adding great Northern beans for bulk, protein, and more magnesium.

Dr. Rude says people who are magnesium deficient are resistant to the bone-beneficial effects of parathyroid hormone and vitamin D, which boost the uptake of calcium and help deposit it in the bone. Other evidence links low magnesium intake with abnormal bone formation, and indicates that magnesium deprivation triggers bone loss.

—Robert K. Rude, M.D., *is professor of medicine at the University of Southern California School of Medicine in Los Angeles.*

DON'T THIN OUT YOUR SKELETON

If you lose too much weight or are natu-rally very thin, you could be at higher risk for osteoporosis.

Think of your bones as levers that help lift limbs. When these levers lift more weight, they become denser and more resistant to fracture. That's why a little meat on your bones can help protect them, says Jane Kirby, R.D. Being too thin is actually a risk factor for osteoporosis.

There's more. Kirby says that when women shed too many pounds and body fat drops dramatically, menstruation ceases and blood estrogen levels plummet. The lack of es-trogen imperils bones, because this hormone helps calcium get into your skeleton and stay there.

To find out where you stand, Kirby recommends taking your Body Mass Index (BMI). BMI compares weight to height to determine proper weight. Here's how.

1. Convert your height to inches.
2. Weigh yourself first thing in the morning, naked.

3. Multiply your weight in pounds by 704.5.

4. Divide #3 by your height in inches.

5. Divide #4 by your height in inches again. That's your BMI.

Below 19 means you are too thin; 19 to 25 translates to a normal weight; 25 to 29.9 means you're overweight; you're obese if your BMI is 30 or above.

If you're underweight, you may need to cut back on exercise so you don't burn more calories than you consume—but enough that you still get the minimum weight-bearing, strength-training, and flexibility quotas described in Schedule Bone Benefiters into Your Day on page 41. You also need to eat more, being sure to choose a balanced diet.

—Jane Kirby, R.D., *is a nutrition consultant in Charlotte, Vermont.*

HAVE AN EGG A DAY

Chances are, you've cracked down on your egg intake in the name of better health. But eggs are good for your bones and may be better for your heart than you might think.

Eggs have taken a beating as promoters of clogged arteries and heart disease. It's the cholesterol thing.

Granted, they do pack a wallop: about 213 milligrams per medium egg. "But let's set the record straight," says Kathleen M. Zelman, R.D. "They contain little saturated fat, the main villain in boosting blood cholesterol concentrations."

In fact, some studies have exonerated eggs from their association with cardiovascular disease. That's good news for your bones. Eggs are rich in bone-building nutrients.

A medium egg supplies a third of your Daily Value for vitamin K, a little-recognized vitamin that's vital to bone density. Eggs also deliver vitamin D, a claim very few foods can make. Vitamin D promotes calcium absorption and helps deliver the mineral to bone.

If your blood cholesterol is within normal range, one egg a day might be just what the doctor ordered for your bones. Just skip the sausage, bacon, cheese, and home fries that drive up saturated fat. And you can't get away with ordering a "white" omelette, because all the bone-boosting vitamins are in the yolk.

—Kathleen M. Zelman, R.D., *is a nutrition consultant in Atlanta and coauthor of* Healthy Eating for Babies and Toddlers.

DON'T FORGET MANGANESE

Talk about obscure. Manganese is a mineral truly living in the shadows, but it has an important role in heading off osteoporosis.

Pity poor manganese. Few people know it even exists, and when they hear about it, it's often confused with another mineral, magnesium. That's probably all right. Both contribute to bone health throughout your lifetime, says Forrest H. Nielsen, Ph.D.

Studies suggest that manganese is needed to form the proper matrix on which calcium is deposited to form bone. There are suspicions that manganese helps prevent calcium losses for women who are past menopause, says Dr. Nielsen.

On the other hand, manganese deficiency could lead to bone abnormalities, he warns. Be sure to get an adequate intake of 2 to 5 milligrams a day.

It makes sense to eat foods rich in manganese, including whole grains, nuts, leafy vegetables, and tea—as well as pineapple, which contains 2.6 grams of manganese per cup of the diced fruit.

This salad stars three manganese-rich foods—pineapples, rice, and almonds—and has more than 8 grams of manganese.

Pineapple-Rice Medley

2½ cups cooked medium-grain brown rice
1 cup chopped pineapple
½ cup raisins
⅓ cup chopped toasted almonds
¼ cup chopped green onions
¼ teaspoon ground allspice
2 tablespoons olive oil
2 tablespoons lime juice

Combine the rice, pineapple, raisins, almonds, onions, allspice, oil, and lime juice in a large bowl and chill before enjoying.

Makes about 4½ cups.

—Forrest H. Nielsen, Ph.D., *is the center director and research nutritionist at the United States Department of Agriculture Grand Forks Human Nutrition Research Center in Grand Forks, North Dakota.*

DISCOVER K-POWER

*The likes of lettuce, kale, spinach,
avocados, and broccoli supply vitamin K,
which might fight off hip fracture when
consumed in adequate amounts.*

A study of 72,327 female nurses over a 10-year period
found that women who ate lettuce at least once a day
were less than half as likely to break a hip than those who
ate lettuce no more than once a week. Researchers credited
vitamin K for these promising results.

According to bone researcher Diane Feskanich, Sc.D.,
little-known vitamin K promotes the chemical conversion of
a specific bone protein known as osteocalcin. Once this
transaction has occurred, osteocalcin can do its job of
strengthening bone tissue.

In other research, people who took vitamin K supplements lost less calcium in their urine and showed better
bone mineral density than people who didn't take vitamin K.
Still other research links low concentrations of vitamin K to
low bone mineral density and bone fractures.

No one knows exactly how much vitamin K it takes to
keep bones healthy and strong, but it could be much more
than the Recommended Dietary Allowance of 65 micrograms for women and 80 micrograms for men (which are set
to stave off blood clotting, not to strengthen bone). Dr. Feskanich's own study suggests that women may need 109 micrograms a day or more to fend off fractures.

The good news is that it's not too hard to get your K if
you eat salad, because it's plentiful in leaf lettuce, endive,
watercress, and spinach. If you don't like greens alone, add
cooked dark greens such as kale or spinach to soups, stews,
omelettes, and frittatas. A mere half-cup of cooked cabbage,

spinach, kale, or collard greens is more than enough to meet the 109 microgram level. Brussels sprouts, broccoli, soybean oil, and whole eggs also supply you with vitamin K.

One caveat: If you take the prescription medication warfarin (Coumadin), ask your doctor before increasing vitamin K. The two work against each other.

—Diane Feskanich, Sc.D., *is a researcher and instructor at Harvard Medical School in Boston.*

MAKE A TOAST TO YOUR BONES

You've probably heard that moderate amounts of alcohol might be good for your heart. Well, it might also be good for your bones.

Although chronic alcohol consumption is likely to weaken bones, moderate alcohol intake does just the opposite, says Diane Feskanich, Sc.D. Her research suggests that postmenopausal women who indulge in five or more drinks a week can actually improve their bones. (A drink is defined as 12 ounces of regular beer, 1.5 ounces of 80-proof liquor, or 5 ounces of wine.)

Women in the study had more than 10 percent higher bone mineral density in their spines than the nondrinkers. The study concludes that moderate alcohol consumption might be beneficial because higher estrogen levels are present in women who consume alcohol, and estrogen is associated with a reduction in bone loss.

This news begs the question: Should you start drinking to build bone tissue? No, says Dr. Feskanich. If you don't like the taste or the effects of alcohol, by all means avoid it. And if you do choose to drink alcohol, know that moderation matters. More is not better, especially since alcohol has been tentatively linked with breast cancer in some women.

—Diane Feskanich, Sc.D., *is a researcher and instructor at Harvard Medical School in Boston.*

BONE UP ON BORON

Boron sounds like the name of a distant planet in another galaxy, but don't be put off by the name. Bones need boron in a big way.

Boron is the strong, silent type. Yet it seems that this mighty trace mineral is poised for stardom, despite its low profile. The evidence that boron is essential to good health is becoming increasingly persuasive, says Forrest H. Nielsen, Ph.D., who suspects that many of us have a boron shortfall.

According to Dr. Nielsen, boron acts like a supporting player in bone health, possibly by increasing the body's uptake of calcium, magnesium, and phosphorus, which are necessary for dense, fracture-free bones.

Boron might be particularly useful for postmenopausal women on estrogen therapy. Studies show that boron might enhance and mimic some effects of supplemental estrogen, which works to enhance bone strength.

All you need is 3 milligrams a day, but it's important you get it. It's not listed on package labels, so here's the word from Dr. Nielsen: Legumes, such as lentils, peas, and peanuts, are boron bonanzas.

A good way to get your boron is to think of throwing beans into prepared dishes such as salads, soups, and stews. Make chili with half the meat and double the beans.

If whole beans aren't your bag, home in on hummus, a garlicy ground chickpea spread. This Middle Eastern favorite makes a good sandwich spread or dip for pitas and vegetables. If you can spare the fat, don't discount good old peanut butter sandwiches as boron boosters, either.

—Forrest H. Nielsen, Ph.D., *is the center director and research nutritionist at the United States Department of Agriculture Grand Forks Human Nutrition Research Center in Grand Forks, North Dakota.*

BE PRUDENT ABOUT PROTEIN

Protein is vital for strength and energy, but too much of it creates calcium loss, compromising bone health.

It's an accepted fact that eating too much protein leaches calcium from the body, jeopardizing bone health. "The question is, how much is too much? And when should you worry?" challenges James C. Fleet, Ph.D.

Many women eat more than the Recommended Dietary Allowance (RDA) of 50 grams daily. Eating excess protein produces an acid load in the body that must be countered by chemicals released from bone tissue, according to Dr. Fleet. In the process, calcium is liberated and washed away in the urine, contributing to bone thinning.

At first glance, animal protein seems to be the villain, since it contains more acid-making amino acids, the building blocks of protein. Yet, Dr. Fleet cautions, the research implicating animal protein, rather than excess protein, may need a second look. "Certain plant foods can produce just as much acid as their animal counterparts," he asserts.

Here's the bottom line. You need protein. It's an integral part of bones. Just don't go overboard. Dr. Fleet says eating twice the RDA for protein in any form boosts daily calcium requirements by a hefty 250 milligrams and could contribute to osteoporosis. Do your bones a favor by eating protein as part of a well-balanced diet that includes 1,500 milligrams of calcium daily.

—James C. Fleet, Ph.D., *is the director of the graduate program in nutrition at the University of North Carolina at Greensboro.*

BUILD COLLAGEN WITH VITAMIN C

It takes more than calcium and vitamin D to build strong bones and keep them that way. Vitamin C actually helps build the very foundation that makes up bone structure.

Vitamin C typically grabs attention as an immune system booster. Still, vitamin C is vastly underrated for its starring role in bone health.

Vitamin C's stimulation of collagen production is arguably its most notable function in bone health, says Deborah E. Kipp, R.D., Ph.D. Collagen is connective tissue that holds together bones (and other body tissues), providing their matrix, or core. This matrix is then fortified by minerals such as calcium and magnesium, providing strength and fracture resistance.

Get the 60 milligrams of vitamin C you need with at least one vitamin C–rich food, such as citrus fruits or juice, every day. Smokers need a daily minimum of 100 milligrams of vitamin C, because cigarettes reduce blood levels, says Dr. Kipp.

Other good sources of vitamin C are strawberries, mango, cantaloupe, kiwifruit, watermelon, and bell pepper. Make an exotic fruit salad, or toss sautéed red bell pepper slices into your spaghetti sauce.

—Deborah E. Kipp, R.D., Ph.D., *is professor of nutrition at the University of North Carolina at Greensboro.*

ORDER SALT OFF YOUR MENU

High salt intake can threaten your bones. But that doesn't mean you have to bypass the drive-thru window. Just make smart menu choices.

It's no wonder that an estimated 75 percent of the sodium in the typical American diet is derived from highly processed foods, such as burgers and pizza. Not only do processed foods contain added sodium as a flavor enhancer but sodium also is used as a preservative, leavening agent, thickener, binder, curing agent, buffer to control acidity, emulsifier, mold inhibitor, and agent in artificial sweeteners.

Plain and simple: The more sodium, the greater the calcium loss, says Robert P. Heaney, M.D. When you can't cook at home and control how much sodium goes into your meals, here are some ways to choose the lowest-sodium options when dining out.

- Avoid ham or sausage breakfast sandwiches and reach instead for a bagel with cream cheese and fruit.
- Opt for broiled chicken with steamed vegetables and new potatoes instead of mashed potatoes and gravy.
- Stroll on by sodium-soaked chicken Caesar salads, heading for the supermarket salad bar instead, where low-sodium vegetables are plentiful.
- Tell your Asian restaurant to hold the "brown sauce" or put it in a separate container where you can be conservative about how much salty soy you use. Tell the restaurant to hold the monosodium glutamate (MSG) flavoring, too. Use more duck sauce and pepper for flavor.
- Go easy on prepared ketchup, mustard, horseradish, and barbecue sauce. Ask for extra tomatoes, lettuce, and onions for garnish instead.

—Robert P. Heaney, M.D., *is John A. Creighton University professor in the department of medicine at Creighton University in Omaha, Nebraska.*

CHOOSE LATTE OVER BLACK COFFEE

The caffeine in coffee can leach precious calcium from your body, weakening bones over time. If you can't stand the thought of giving up your java, here's how you can enjoy it, guilt-free.

Rather than ordering your morning brew black, go for a latte or a cappuccino. The added milk can help cut the losses of calcium you are causing by drinking caffeinated beverages.

As a general rule, compensate for every cup of coffee by drinking three glasses of milk, says Linda K. Massey, R.D., Ph.D. Frothed-top javas get you off to a good start.

To protect your calcium intake, limit your coffee consumption to 16 ounces a day, she adds.

Of course, it's best to simply moderate your caffeine consumption. If you love the taste of coffee or spend a lot of time around coffeehouses, switch to decaf—or at least half decaf mixed with half regular.

—Linda K. Massey, R.D., Ph.D., *is professor of human nutrition at Washington State University in Spokane, Washington.*

GO FISH

*Fish harbors a type of fat that fosters
skeletal strength. Are you getting enough?
You might need to get in the swim.*

If you're like most people, you work hard to hold back on
fat to foster weight control and head off heart disease. But
don't forget that your bones can benefit from certain fats,
says Bruce A. Watkins, Ph.D.

Dr. Watkins is an advocate of eating omega-3 fatty acids.
In one study, animals that ate omega-3 fatty acids produced
more new bone proteins, which provide the basis for mineralization. Mineralization occurs when your body lays down
the likes of calcium, phosphorus, and magnesium to boost
bone density, reducing the threat of osteoporosis later in life.

According to Dr. Watkins, fish is the food chain's primary food source of omega-3's. All seafood is beneficial, but
the fattier the fish, the better the omega-3 source. That
makes salmon, sardines, anchovies, bluefish, mackerel, her-
ring, and trout especially good for bones, he says. Eating the
soft bones of sardines and anchovies increases calcium intake, too.

If you're still worried about your heart, you may be
heartened to know that omega-3's are the "good fats" that
help keep cholesterol and triglyceride levels in check while
defeating blood clots, Dr. Watkins adds.

The government hasn't set a recommended daily
amount for omega-3's yet, but a few fish dinners a week are
likely beneficial, says Dr. Watkins.

—Bruce A. Watkins, Ph.D., *is professor of nutrition in
the department of food science at Purdue University in West
Lafayette, Indiana.*

The Sooner You Start, the Better

Your children's needs for calcium and other bone-forming nutrients might be even greater than yours. Fill your refrigerator with food that they—and everyone's bones—will like. The whole family will benefit.

Childhood is a time of tremendous bone growth, says Kathleen M. Zelman, R.D. Calcium needs increase to 1,300 milligrams a day from ages 9 to 18, up from the 800 milligrams that children need daily from ages 4 through 8.

Calcium requirements reach their peak during adolescence, yet many adolescents have inadequate calcium intakes—perhaps because this is when many teenage girls stop drinking milk.

Here is some grab food that makes it easy for your children, not to mention yourself, to consume calcium and its supporting nutrients.

- Homemade popsicles from calcium-enriched orange juice
- Presliced and precleaned carrot sticks and other vegetables, with an herb-yogurt dip on the side
- Small containers of cottage cheese with some small cans of pineapple or peaches that they can mix in
- Cubed hard cheese and whole-grain crackers
- Eggs, so they can make a quick microwave scramble

- Easy snack bars or party mixes, made from their favorite whole-grain cereal or granola, with their favorite nuts, spices, and dried fruit (follow the directions on cereal boxes)
- Premade peanut butter sandwiches

—Kathleen M. Zelman, R.D., *is a nutrition consultant in Atlanta and coauthor of* Healthy Eating for Babies and Toddlers.

TREAT YOUR INNER ARCHITECTURE TO TOFU

Once relegated to the realm of health-nut fare, tofu is now front and center in the supermarket. One of the reasons for its popularity is that the word is out—the nutrients in those silky white blocks are kind to your bones.

Every time you turn around, health experts are trumpeting the benefits of soy.

"You can hardly ignore soy," says Evelyn Tribole, R.D. And you shouldn't. Soy foods reduce blood cholesterol, mitigate menopausal symptoms, help fight cancerous tumors, combat dangerous blood clots, keep blood vessels elastic—and yes, tofu might also boost bone health.

Soy foods contain isoflavones, plant substances thought to be responsible for building bone. Tofu is a convenient source of isoflavones—neutral enough to sneak its way into many meals as a hidden supplement or a creamy base, or to star as the main protein source.

Tofu can also be a tremendous calcium source. To get the most calcium, Tribole says you should always purchase tofu processed with calcium sulfate, which is readily available from major brands. A half-block of firm tofu prepared with calcium sulfate holds a whopping 861 grams of calcium—nearly a full day's needs.

Here are some ways to introduce the silky blocks into your diet.

- Marinate a slab of extra-firm tofu (with twice the calcium of the softer varieties) and toss it on the grill.
- Replace one-third to one-half the amount of cream cheese with pureed tofu in cheesecake recipes.
- Stir-fry tofu with vegetables such as broccoli, asparagus, and red bell pepper to serve over rice.
- For a dip, blend pureed tofu instead of sour cream in with your favorite dried soup mix, such as onion.
- Buy chocolate, cappuccino, or butterscotch instant tofu pudding mixes (such as the Mori-Nu brand) at the health food store. It's sinfully rich, and as simple as whipping a block of tofu and a pack of pudding flavor mix in your blender.

—Evelyn Tribole, R.D., *is a nutrition consultant in Irvine, California, and author of* Healthy Homestyle Cooking.

CONSIDER ISOFLAVONE SUPPLEMENTS

Do you want soy's estrogen-like benefits but don't like tofu or soy milk? You'll be pleased to know that isoflavones—soy's bone-boosting ingredient—come in pill form.

As you know, when estrogen levels drop, your risk for osteoporosis rises. If your estrogen levels are dwindling because of menopause and you're not on estrogen-replacement therapy, isoflavone supplements can help boost your hormone levels, says Densie L. Webb, R.D., Ph.D.

Start by taking 30 milligrams and work up to 50 milligrams a day—which is the equivalent of two daily servings of soy foods.

Dr. Webb says that no one knows whether it's safe to take isoflavone pills if you're also undergoing hormone-replacement therapy, because it mimics some of the effects of isoflavones in the body. Your best bet is to check with your doctor before popping isoflavone pills, advises Dr. Webb, especially if you have a history of breast cancer.

—Densie L. Webb, R.D., Ph.D., *is a nutrition consultant in Austin, Texas.*

KEEP KIDNEY STONES AWAY

It's a double-edged sword—calcium can cause kidney stones, but your bones can't do without it.

They may be relatively small, but kidney stones are a big pain. Think of a rough pebble making its way down a narrow passage well-constructed to carry a stream of urine, but hardly designed to carry a calcified object.

Sound like a plumbing problem? Well, if so, deal with it like one.

Essentially, adding extra fluid can dilute and break down the "clog." According to Linda K. Massey, R.D., Ph.D., drinking eight 8-ounce glasses of water will minimize the risk of kidney stones by diluting calcium concentrations in the urine.

Other than drinking plenty of liquids, you can also monitor calcium intake. The object is to be sure to get your daily quota, but don't exceed 2,000 milligrams.

—Linda K. Massey, R.D., Ph.D., *is professor of human nutrition at Washington State University in Spokane, Washington.*

Skeletal Strength through Exercise

"The best exercises are whatever you like to do and what you'll continue doing."

—Felicia Cosman, M.D.,
osteoporosis specialist and endocrinologist, clinical research center of Helen Hayes Hospital, West Haverstraw, New York

SCHEDULE BONE BENEFITERS INTO YOUR DAY

Your own body is your most valuable and economical piece of equipment when it comes to preserving bone through exercise. Do it every day.

A lifestyle that includes a broad spectrum of exercises will give you the best chance of stopping and reversing bone loss as well as keep you fit enough to avoid injury.

There's no perfect better-bones exercise blueprint, but experts generally agree that you need to exercise *regularly*, and that your bones benefit from a *variety* of activities. The cornerstone of your exercise routine should involve weight-bearing activities supplemented with strength, flexibility, and balance training—although no comparative studies have been done regarding the ideal ratio, says Felicia Cosman, M.D.

Make exercise a habit, like brushing your teeth, not something you do when you want to fit into a bathing suit. And once you start, don't stop, because any bone loss you were staving off will ensue quickly. To ensure that you get a balanced week of regular exercise, try scheduling your workouts in a daily planner.

Dr. Cosman recommends a schedule consisting of a minimum of the following activities.

Weight-Bearing Aerobic Activity—30 minutes, three times a week. Walking, running, dancing, aerobics, and jumping rope are all examples of good weight-bearing exercises because you move your entire body, without having your weight supported by a bicycle or water, for example.

Gravity causes your body to land with an impact, and your muscles pull on your bones. Not only has this type of resistance of the Earth on your skeleton been found to slow bone loss but it also shows promise for *new* bone growth.

Strength Training—15 minutes, three times a week. Statistically, people with higher muscle mass are less susceptible to osteoporosis. It only makes sense, because bone is stimulated when muscles contract. The importance of strength training in bone health was reinforced by a study conducted at Tufts University in Boston, where doctors found that women who performed strength-training exercises not only became stronger but also gained bone and improved their balance and flexibility.

Lifting weights, or using strength-training machines, strengthens bones all over your body, especially if you exercise the major muscle groups in your legs, arms, and trunk. Just be sure to start out at a low weight that you can lift 15 times in a row. Gradually build up to heavier weights.

Balance and Flexibility—5 to 10 minutes, three times a week. Balance and flexibility are essential for women with osteoporosis concerns, because as these functions improve, the risk for falls and fractures decreases. In other words, when you're limber and stable, you're less likely to lose your balance and more likely to catch yourself if you trip.

You don't have to be able to swing on a trapeze or twist yourself into a pretzel, but participating in a yoga or tai chi class once a week, or just doing a simple stretch routine first thing in the morning, will put some balance into your life.

If you have bone problems such as arthritis or osteoporosis, know your limits. "Rather than high-impact exercises such as running and aerobics, opt for low-impact exercise if you experience pain or if you've had compression fractures. If you have any osteoporotic problems, don't do exercises that involve twisting. Most people can do modified forms of strength, flexibility, and balance training," Dr. Cosman says.

—Felicia Cosman, M.D., *is an osteoporosis specialist and endocrinologist at the clinical research center of Helen Hayes Hospital in West Haverstraw, New York.*

FIND HIDDEN EXERCISE OPPORTUNITIES

Wouldn't be caught dead in spandex? That's okay—you can stay in denim and as far away from the gym as your back-yard. It's not as hard as you think to get the exercise you need. Everyday activi-ties can contribute to bone building.

Today's conveniences mean people don't have to churn butter, work in the field, and chop wood anymore, but that doesn't mean you can't get exercise from modern-day living. "You don't have to live like people did 100 years ago to have a physically active lifestyle," says Robert Recker, M.D.

If you're able, tote your own groceries and carry home your dry cleaning. Try muscle-moving alternatives to chores like raking the lawn instead of hauling out the leaf blower, or hanging out your laundry. Build up a sweat weeding your garden and transplanting plants. Eliminate couch potato conveniences like the television remote control and garage door opener, advises Dr. Recker.

Count these activities in your exercise log, and exercise won't seem like such a rigid routine. You can log moving boxes in the attic as a strength builder, for example, and washing windows as balance and flexibility training for the day.

If your job is sedentary or you're stuck in an office all day, there are still ways to sneak in exercise. For example, walk down the hall to deliver a message to a coworker instead of sending an e-mail. When you're waiting at the copy machine, do some stretches. And no matter what floor you work on, forgo the elevator for the stairs.

—Robert Recker, M.D., *is the director of the osteoporosis research center at the Creighton University School of Medicine in Omaha, Nebraska.*

SWING INTO SHAPE

You might think that dancing is too much fun to count as exercise . . . but it does.

Forget the excuses. You have two left feet. . . were left by the punch bowl at the prom. . . have no sense of rhythm. . . or don't know any steps. Get onto the dance floor anyway and start moving your arms, hips, and feet!

No matter how you do it, dancing is a perfectly acceptable way to add some bop to your bone health program because it's a weight-bearing exercise that staves off bone density loss, says Joseph Lane, M.D. And it's never too late to develop a little coordination, which you're going to need as your risk of fall-related fractures increases with age.

Viennese researchers observed the bone-mass density of women with osteoporosis who participated in a dancing group approximately 3 hours a week. Over the course of a year, they showed an increase in bone density in their spines.

"You need a broad spectrum of exercise to develop your coordination and balance," says Dr. Lane, and that includes dancing. So whether it's line dancing, polka, fox trot, boogie, or freestylin', 30 minutes on the dance floor 3 or 4 days a week can be a swinging way to keep weak bones at bay.

Can't get to the dance floor? Turn on the radio or put your favorite hip hop on the stereo and start moving to your own beat.

—Joseph Lane, M.D., *is professor of orthopaedic surgery at Weill Medical College of Cornell University and chief of the metabolic bone disease department at the Hospital for Special Surgery, both in New York City.*

STEP FORWARD TO REVERSE BONE LOSS

Almost anyone can do it, and the results give you all-around protection against bone loss. Whatever way you look at it, walking might be the best thing for you.

The importance of walking to bone health is overwhelming. In one study, people with osteoporosis who walked more than 30 minutes a day experienced less deformity in their spines than their counterparts who didn't walk. Other studies show that walking helps improve balance and coordination—and reduces the risk of falling in older adults. Research also shows that walkers experience significantly less bone loss in their leg bones than nonwalkers.

As a weight-bearing activity, brisk walking is superior, says Roberto Civitelli, M.D. It's not jarring to your joints and muscles like jogging or jumping rope, but your whole skeleton still takes the impact of your body weight as you step. This is called loading, and it's what stimulates bone formation and also strengthens your backbone, he adds.

For example, a year-long study of postmenopausal female walkers conducted by the Jean Meyer Human Nutrition Research Center on Aging at Tufts University in Boston indicated that walkers have up to 7 years more bone in reserve than nonwalkers. At any age (the average age was 62), the women who walked more than a mile a day had 4 percent more bone density overall compared to women who didn't walk a mile.

If you're overweight, out of shape, or new to exercise, start with a slow pace (about 3 miles per hour). As you improve, vary your routine by adding hills or increasing your pace. Remember to breathe, walk tall, and watch your step!

A half-hour to an hour of walking, three or four times a week, is needed to reap the maximum bone and back benefits, Dr. Civitelli explains.

—Roberto Civitelli, M.D., *is associate professor in the department of bone and mineral diseases at Washington University's Barnes-Jewish Hospital in St. Louis.*

ROAM THE MALL

If you're like many women who've never exercised, and you're reluctant to start, mall walking can get you—and keep you—motivated.

Your local shopping arena is a fun setting to catch up with old friends and make new ones, while walking into better bones. A study conducted at the University of Iowa found that older women who exercised regularly considered physical activity a part of their social lives, not something apart from it.

Not only are malls very social places but they also offer protection from the elements, a secure and well-lit environment, and ever-changing surroundings. "People tend to stick with exercise programs if there's an incentive or it's enjoyable," says Margaret Burghardt, M.D.

Many malls open their doors to walkers before they're open to the general public. Call your local mall to inquire about walking hours. Some communities also have walking clubs that provide free log sheets and gifts for achieving your goals.

Of course, you have to remember that this is an exercise program, not a shopping program—so keep moving past the sale advertisements, and that goes for the gooey cinnamon rolls, too!

—Margaret Burghardt, M.D., *is a staff physician in primary care sports medicine at the University of Western Ontario in London, Canada.*

ADD WEIGHT
TO YOUR WALK

A walking program with wrist and body weights makes a big impact on keeping you strong, solid, and safe.

Valerie Weil, M.D., suggests wearing soft 1- to 3-pound wrist weights when you go for a walk. Activating your arms adds extra oomph to the weight-bearing benefits of walking, which means an increase in skeletal loading (the impact of your body weight that helps generate bone). It also strengthens your arms, not to mention enhancing the cardiovascular component of your workout.

Don't wear these weights while running or doing aerobics, though, she says, because they can increase the risk of ligament injury or stress fractures.

Weighted vests are another way to add some resistance training to your exercise program. In a study at the University of Utah, women who participated in a 9-month program where they used increasingly heavier resistance with a weighted vest showed significant improvement in lower-body strength and muscle power over women in a control group. Due to the women's improved overall fitness, researchers also concluded that walking with the weighted vest could reduce the risk of falling for postmenopausal women.

There are numerous vests on the market that can be adjusted to different weights. Purchase wrist weights and weighted vests from sporting goods suppliers or fitness stores.

—Valerie Weil, M.D., *is assistant professor of medicine at the Hospital of the University of Pennsylvania in Philadelphia.*

RESHAPE YOUR BACK

Whether your back has started to sway too much or it's hunching you over, the pelvic tilt can help correct either extreme—and bring relief in the process.

The backbone is the region of most concern for people with osteoporosis. When the bones soften enough, you can develop a vertebral compression fracture simply by sneezing, which can lead to a lifetime of pain and reduced mobility.

These fractures, often coupled with weak back muscles, create kyphosis, the posture marked by rolled-forward shoulders and a humped back (sometimes known as dowager's hump). Poor posture increases the risk of falling, which increases the chances for further deformity and even fatal injury.

What can be done to avoid this downward spiral? A Mayo Clinic study found significant improvement in severe kyphosis, or humpback posture, in women who increased the strength of their back muscles over a 2-year period. Another Mayo Clinic study on women with osteoporosis concluded that the risk of vertebral fractures is likely to decrease after strengthening back muscles.

Just be choosy about what you do to strengthen your back, because people with osteoporosis can't always do the same workout as their stronger-boned sisters and brothers, advises Robert Uebele, P.T. Yoga has some great strengthening poses, for example, but the ones where you arch your back while on your hands and knees—or twist your torso sharply to one side while seated—might not be for you.

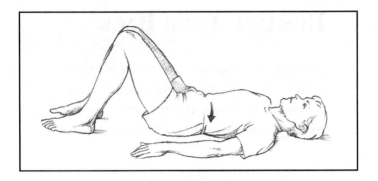

The pelvic tilt is a gentle starting point for strengthening your back. In the long run, it can help correct a swayback or humpback posture, and in the short run, it might relieve pain from sitting too long.

Lie on your back with your knees bent. To get comfortable, you can place a flat pillow under your head and a rolled-up towel under your neck for support. Inhale fully, letting your chest and belly expand. As you exhale, flatten the small of your back into the floor by tightening your stomach muscles (imagine curling your tailbone into your navel). Inhale deeply into your abdomen again, and repeat the curl as you exhale. Repeat this a few times, until you feel your back muscles loosen and relax. To sit up, roll to one side and push yourself up with your hands.

You can do this exercise just about anywhere, in just a few minutes. It might be the most productive time you ever spend lying on the ground.

—Robert Uebele, P.T., *is the clinical coordinator for the rehabilitation unit at Bayhealth Medical Center in Milford, Delaware.*

RUN *RIGHT* TO REDUCE YOUR RISK

Running is great for bone-building benefits—but only when you start out on the right foot.

If you're interested in starting a running program or progressing from walking to running, do it slowly and take precautions. Otherwise, you risk damaging rather than helping your bones.

"Running is a great weight-bearing exercise," says osteoporosis expert Michael DiMuzio, Ph.D. "I don't recommend, however, that people go from doing nothing to logging miles without knowing what they're doing, because then you're actually raising the possibility of developing osteoarthritis and injury."

For example, running on asphalt and wearing the wrong shoes might put too much stress on your joints and bones, while running on broken sidewalks increases your risk of falling, cautions Dr. DiMuzio. Wear a well-cushioned pair of running shoes and confine your workouts to either a track or a soft running surface like dirt.

Running too fast before you're ready can also make you dizzy and overfatigued, making you susceptible to falling. The following introductory guideline is recommended by the American Council on Exercise: Walk 50 yards, then jog the next 50 yards, and repeat this interval 10 to 20 times for no more than 30 minutes for the first month. Gradually increase your jogging intervals to 2 or more miles.

Be sure to allow 1 day of rest between your workouts so your body can recover. Both novices and experienced runners should perform warmup and cooldown exercises.

—Michael DiMuzio, Ph.D., *is the director of the osteoporosis prevention and research center at the Highland Park Hospital in Highland Park, Illinois.*

DON'T RUN INTO TROUBLE

Training so hard that your period stops is a dangerous sign that you shouldn't ignore, because it can send you down the road to osteoporosis.

R unning hard can be good for your bones if you're in shape and don't have joint problems, but taken to an extreme, it can lead to unexpected trouble.

Amenorrhea, the cessation of your menstrual period, can set in when your body fat drops below a critical percentage, says John Turco, M.D. This kind of risk is high among teenagers, women in their twenties, and some competitive athletes, rather than in older women, who usually have a higher percentage of body fat to begin with.

Excessive exercise isn't the only cause of amenorrhea, says Dr. Turco, but it's definitely one of the major ones. But whatever the cause, the consequences are the same. Just as for a woman in menopause, when your period stops, the estrogen that protects against bone loss dwindles. So at the very age when you should be building bone mass, you could be losing it instead.

The bottom line, notes Dr. Turco, is that if you run to such extremes that your period stops, quit running. Cut back on your workouts. If your period doesn't return in a few months, consult your doctor.

—John Turco, M.D., *is associate professor of clinical medicine at Dartmouth Medical School in Hanover, New Hampshire.*

TENNIS, ANYONE?

Think running is the winner when it comes to bone-building exercise? Well, guess again. Tennis is the winner, hands down.

A study conducted by the department of rheumatology at St. Thomas' Hospital in London found that female tennis players ages 40 to 65 had greater bone mass in their spines, necks, and forearms than women who didn't play tennis. In fact, the tennis players had greater overall bone mineral density than even female runners in the same study group.

"Putting stress on your bones is one of the key elements in preventing bone loss," says Michael DiMuzio, Ph.D., "and playing tennis puts stress on your entire skeleton because you're on your legs moving all over the court."

If you love tennis, aim for 1 hour of tennis a week to obtain its weight-bearing benefits. Invite a friend to play with you, and you can do some bone-building "lobbing" together.

—Michael DiMuzio, Ph.D., *is the director of the osteoporosis prevention and research center at the Highland Park Hospital in Highland Park, Illinois.*

GO WITH THE FLOW

The slow, fluid movements of tai chi will give you the benefit of peace of mind— but they'll also give you the benefit of better bones.

Tai chi is a martial art developed 700 years ago in China. If you practice this discipline, which stresses mental focus and proper body alignment, you'll also be doing your bones a great service, says tai chi instructor Tricia Yu.

"Tai chi is a weight-bearing exercise, but because it uses slow, gentle movements, there's very little risk for injuries," she says. Yu suggests the following beginner's exercise, which she calls Crane Takes Flight, for strengthening and stretching your quadriceps and back every day.

1. Stand with your feet parallel and shoulder-width apart, toes pointing forward. Your weight should be evenly distributed over both feet. (If you're unsure of your balance, stand next to a wall or chair for support.)

2. Bend your knees, keeping them lined up with your feet. Keep your posture straight and let your arms hang at your sides.

3. As you breathe in, slowly straighten your knees and bring your arms up to shoulder height as though you're making a snow angel.

4. Slowly return your arms to your sides as you breathe out.

5. Repeat four more times.

—Tricia Yu *is a tai chi instructor in Madison, Wisconsin, and author of* T'ai Chi Fundamentals for Health Professionals and Instructors.

TAKE A SPIN

Looking for a bone-building exercise that works like a breeze? Then get out that old bicycle and go for a ride.

Putting some pedaling back in your life is good for the bones. Even though cycling isn't considered a weight-bearing exercise, it has benefits that are similar to walking or running.

"Cycling uses muscle groups that put stress on the bones, like the quadriceps, hamstrings, and calf muscles. There's also some degree of trunk stability involved on a bike, so you're also using your back," says Margaret Burghardt, M.D. All the pulling it takes to ride actually stimulates bone growth as well as strengthens your muscles.

Adjust the seat for outdoor and stationary bicycles so that there's a slight bend in your knee on the downstroke and so that you're leaning slightly forward toward the handlebars.

Stationary cycling can be a safe alternative when the weather is bad or if you're reluctant to take to the streets. But when you're outside, remember to wear a helmet no matter how far or fast you ride, Dr. Burghardt cautions.

—Margaret Burghardt, M.D., *is a staff physician in primary care sports medicine at the University of Western Ontario in London, Canada.*

SEEK FUN AND GAMES

You don't have to be a jock or even have any experience to enjoy playing a sport. In fact, you'll probably have so much fun you'll forget how good it is for you.

Obvious reasons to play sports are because you enjoy teamwork, or you hope to burn extra calories. Here's another—sports also contribute to bone health and coordination, says Felicia Cosman, M.D.

So if you find walking by yourself boring and the gym intimidating, consider playing a game. Research shows that when you find an activity enjoyable, you're more likely to participate on a regular basis. It's the positive social interaction in games like soccer, softball, and basketball that keeps many young girls and women involved in sports, according to Dr. Cosman.

Call your local YMCA/YWCA or your local parks and recreation department for information about sports teams in your area. Don't be shy about asking if anyone wants to get together to play your favorite sport at your work, church, community pool, or neighborhood—even if all of you have different levels of experience, you all get to move.

Let your active children motivate you. If your children are on teams, don't sit on the sidelines. Get up and jog around the field, or shoot some hoops at half-time. You might even form a team for moms or dads.

—**Felicia Cosman, M.D.,** *is an osteoporosis specialist and endocrinologist with the clinical research center of Helen Hayes Hospital in West Haverstraw, New York.*

GET HIP TO STRENGTH

It might seem that our hips can never be thin enough, but when it comes to bones, they can never be strong enough.

Exercise that works your hips is very important to include in your strength-training program, because hips are a common site for osteoporotic fractures, says Miriam Nelson, Ph.D.

Try Dr. Nelson's hip-extension exercise to strengthen and tighten your hamstrings (thighs) and gluteus maximus (backside). Perform this exercise two or three times per week starting with 3- to 5-pound ankle weights (if you're able). Remember to stay relaxed. Don't lock your knees or tighten your back.

1. Stand behind a chair and grasp it for support, keeping your toes pointed forward.

2. Bend forward 45° at the waist, keeping your legs straight and perpendicular to the floor.

3. Slowly lift your right leg straight up behind you, keeping your foot flexed until it forms a straight line with your back.

4. Pause for a breath and slowly lower your leg to the starting position. Alternate legs until you have done eight lifts on each side. Rest for 2 minutes and then repeat the set.

—Miriam Nelson, Ph.D., *is the director of the center for physical fitness and assistant professor of nutrition at Tufts University in Boston, and author of the best-selling book,* Strong Women Stay Young.

JOIN THE QUAD SQUAD

Whether you're 25 or 85, you'll benefit from working your upper leg muscles.

Getting out of a chair and playing basketball don't appear to be very similar, until you realize that they both rely on the quadriceps muscles in the front of your thighs. So it makes sense to keep these muscles strong to accomplish what you want to, at whatever stage in life you're in. "Besides, we know that progressive strength training has a positive effect on bone at any age," notes Miriam Nelson, Ph.D. An added benefit: toned legs!

Dr. Nelson recommends a knee-extension exercise two to three times a week with 3- to 5-pound weights.

1. Sit in a chair with a deep seat, with your feet shoulder-width apart and your hands resting on your legs or holding the side of the chair. Put a folded towel under your knees for padding, and make sure your knees don't touch each other.

2. Slowly raise your right leg until it is as straight as possible, keeping your foot flexed.

3. Pause for a breath and slowly lower your leg to the starting position.

4. Repeat with your left leg. Alternate until you've completed eight knee extensions with each leg. Rest for 2 minutes and do another set of eight.

—Miriam Nelson, Ph.D., *is the director of the center for physical fitness and assistant professor of nutrition at Tufts University in Boston, and author of the best-selling book,* Strong Women Stay Young.

GET STRONG ABS WITHOUT THE CRUNCH

Don't let spine problems stop you from working out your abdominal region. Try this modified situp.

If you've already suffered a compression fracture or have chronic back pain, you've probably been told to avoid exercises that tend to curve your back, such as situps or toe-touches.

"These kinds of movements put too much compressive force on the spine and can increase the risk of further compression fractures," says Felicia Cosman, M.D. "Even if you haven't suffered a vertebral compression fracture, you should avoid these kinds of activities if you have osteoporosis."

It's important to keep your stomach and abdominal muscles strong, however, because they help stabilize your spine. So how do you do this without "crunching"? Try a modified situp that focuses on tightening your abdominal muscles without curving your back.

1. Lie on the floor or your bed with your knees bent and place your hands on your abdomen.

2. Inhale and tighten your abdominal muscles for a count of three.

3. Exhale and relax for a count of three and repeat 10 times. This exercise can be done every day.

—**Felicia Cosman, M.D.,** *is an osteoporosis specialist and endocrinologist at the clinical research center of Helen Hayes Hospital in West Haverstraw, New York.*

REDUCE RISK TO YOUR WRISTS

When it comes to opening up a jar of peanut butter, keeping your forearms and wrists strong comes in handy. When it comes to preventing osteoporotic injuries, keeping them strong is vital.

Wrists are a primary fracture risk site in women with osteoporosis because they take the brunt of falls, says research physiologist Barbara Drinkwater, Ph.D.

These wrist-curl exercises will help strengthen your forearms as well as improve your grip, giving you a nice advantage if you play a racquet sport or golf. Start with 2- to 5-pound wrist weights or dumbbells.

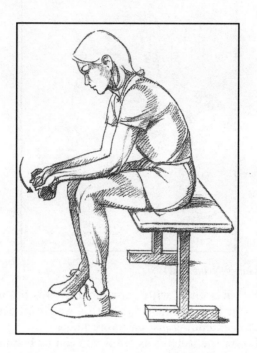

Wrist Curl

1. Sit on a chair with your forearms resting on your thighs, your hands palms up with a weight in each, and your wrists extending just past your knees.

2. Lower the weights by bending your wrists and letting your hands fall back toward your knees. Lift the dumbbells back up and repeat. Start with 4 or 5 repetitions and work your way up to 20. Add a second and third set in subsequent workouts.

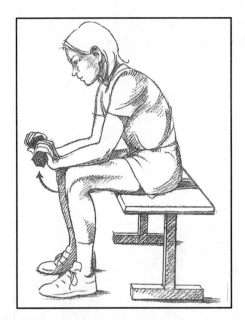

Reverse Wrist Curl

1. Sit on a chair with your forearms resting on your thighs, your hands palm down with a weight in each, and your wrists extending just past your knees.

2. Lower the weights as far as you can by bending your wrists. Lift the weights back up, keeping your forearms in contact with your thighs. Start with 4 or 5 repetitions and work your way up to 20. Add a second and third set in subsequent workouts.

When performing both of these exercises, you'll notice that you have to bend slightly forward to keep your forearms on your thighs. Be sure to keep your back straight by bending at the waist and not letting your back round forward.

—Barbara Drinkwater, Ph.D., *is a research physiologist at Pacific Medical Center in Seattle.*

SPLASH INTO FITNESS

The buoyancy of water makes it a poor medium for weight-bearing exercise, but don't let that persuade you to throw in the towel. Water activities can give you the resistance workout you need without the risk of injury.

Water resistance strengthens and relaxes your muscles. It's a great way to condition yourself for more strenuous exercise, augment your weight-bearing program, or provide a change of scene when bad weather threatens your walking routine, says Roberto Civitelli, M.D.

People who have mobility problems and osteoporotic fractures benefit from swimming or water exercise because of the reduced risk of pain or injury.

Don't think you have to do laps to benefit from the water's resistance, either. Call your community pool to inquire about water aerobics classes, a water volleyball team, or a scuba diving course. Organize a good old Marco Polo game or greased watermelon contest at your next swim party.

Simply *walking* in a pool can be beneficial for those who are overweight, frail, or elderly, because it alleviates pressure on joints while at the same time strengthening leg muscles, says Dr. Civitelli.

—Roberto Civitelli, M.D., *is associate professor in the department of bone and mineral diseases at Washington University's Barnes-Jewish Hospital in St. Louis.*

STRETCHING PUTS SAFETY FIRST

It's not just a prelude to exercise. Get into the habit of stretching your legs every day, and you'll have a surer step.

As we age, we lose our pull—or flexibility—which threatens our balance and increases the risk of falling. Because we walk every day, Robert Whipple, P.T., emphasizes the importance of doing leg stretches. Get more limber, and you'll improve your form in everyday activities, whether it's playing a sport or going down a tricky set of stairs.

When you're about to begin any lower-body workout, such as hiking or jogging, it's essential to loosen up your leg muscles before and after you exercise. Not only are stiff muscles and tendons more likely to become torn or strained, but you also lose alignment when a loose muscle has to compensate for a stiffer one. Stretching will increase blood circulation in your leg muscles and ready them for activity in their most limber state.

The following leg stretches should be done before and after any lower-body workout, especially running and walking.

Calf and Groin Stretch

1. Stand in front of a wall, placing your forearms against it and leaning forward. Rest your head on your hands.

2. Separate your feet from front to back as though you're taking a step toward the wall.

3. Gradually shift your weight forward toward the front leg, letting the front knee bend and extending the back leg behind you.

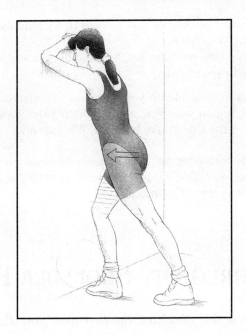

4. Keep your torso vertical as you stretch, with your lower back flat, in order to stretch your groin. (If you've had a hip replacement, however, allow your torso to angle forward, in line with your rear leg.)

5. Hold for 1 minute while breathing regularly. Then repeat with the other leg. For a deeper stretch, increase the distance between your feet; the larger the foot spread from front to back, the more stretch you'll get.

Quad Stretch

1. Standing in front of a wall or sturdy chair for support, bend your right knee, and grab your right foot with your right hand.

2. Pull your foot up so that your heel presses as close

against your buttocks as you can get it, without forcing it. Don't sway your back.

3. Hold this position for 30 seconds, then repeat this stretch with your left leg.

If you're unstable on your feet, do this stretch on the floor by lying on your side and employing the leg and arm opposite to the side you're lying on, Whipple adds.

—Robert Whipple, P.T., *is assistant professor in the department of neurology at the University of Connecticut's health center in Farmington.*

SHRUG OFF SHOULDER PAIN

If you felt pinching the last time you did the wave at a ball game—or had to decline apple picking because of stiff shoulders this year—you're missing some of life's delicious pleasures. Take up shoulder stretches to maintain your mobility—and your fun-loving spirit.

As we age, we lose not only strength in our upper body but also our range of motion, making it difficult to do things like fasten bra snaps, retrieve the mixing bowl from the top shelf, or catch fireflies. Keeping yourself more limber will keep you more active and self-sufficient and lessen your risk of injuries that can be complicated by soft bones.

To stretch your shoulders and chest, physical therapist Robert Whipple recommends the following stretches. "If you haven't done this type of exercise before, you'll probably get some mild strengthening of the muscles in your shoulder joints in the bargain," he adds.

The Wing Back

1. Place your fingers behind your head and point your elbows out to the sides.

2. Slowly pull your elbows farther apart toward the back as far as you can, feeling a strong contraction between your shoulder blades, and hold for 1 minute. Be sure to breathe.

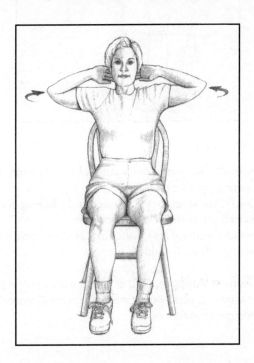

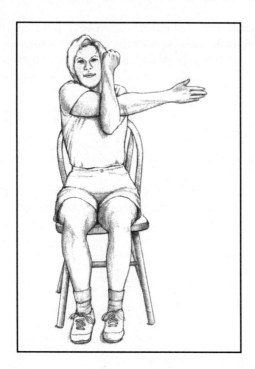

The Wrangler

1. Stretch one arm across your chest, placing it in the bend of your opposite elbow.

2. Hold this stretch for 30 seconds before switching arms. Do two repetitions with each arm.

3. Avoid slumping and slouching. Instead, think of yourself as sitting tall on a saddle.

—Robert Whipple, P.T., *is assistant professor in the department of neurology at the University of Connecticut's health center in Farmington.*

STAND LIKE A WARRIOR

You'll be as proud as a warrior of the strength developing in your hips and legs if you regularly hold yoga poses. And you'll be harder than a warrior to knock down as you get more stable on your feet.

You might think of a yoga session as free-flowing movements, stretches sitting on the floor, and breathing exercises. True, but it also involves striking positions in which you jump or step your legs apart, and then stretch into a lunge or bending pose, which is held for a challenging amount of time.

To hold these standing poses, called asanas, you must completely engage your leg muscles. You also lengthen and release tension in your spine and neck, spread all your toes, and press into all four corners of your feet. This adds up to enhanced strength, flexibility, concentration, and stability.

Ashtanga yoga teacher and personal trainer Tom McCook particularly recommends the standing pose called the proud warrior, since it greatly strengthens your hips and thighs while improving your balance and flexibility.

1. Jump or step your legs 4 feet apart, with your arms extended to the sides, wrists down. Imagine a bar from the top of your head down through the center of your torso to your tailbone. Maintain an awareness of this bar lifting you up as you turn your left foot in and your right foot out.

2. Exhale and bend your right knee to a 90-degree angle if you can, without lunging your knee past your ankle. If you can't bend 90 degrees, bend as far as you can. Try to stretch the right inner thigh muscle toward the right knee while turning the knee slightly to the right.

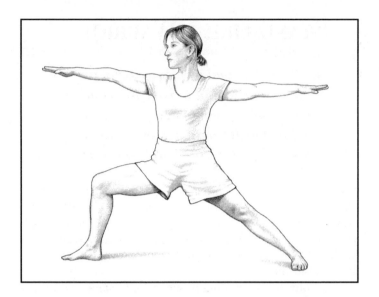

3. Stretch your left leg straight behind you with your foot still turned out, pushing your heel into the floor but not locking your knees. If you start to feel unsure of your balance, stand in a doorway so that you can hold on to the doorjamb.

4. Keep your trunk vertical and facing forward while you look out over your right hand. Both arms should be actively stretching away from each other, even the fingertips, but try to relax the back of your shoulders.

5. Take 5 to 10 breaths as you lunge even lower, continuing to keep your trunk vertical (as if being pulled up by the imaginary bar). Take 5 to 10 breaths here, and then again after you return to your starting position. After three or four lunges, repeat on the other side.

—Tom McCook *is an ACSM personal trainer, Ashtanga yoga teacher, certified Pilates instructor, certified Shiatsu therapist, and founder and director of the Center of Balance in Mountain View, California.*

GET MOVING WITH MAN'S BEST FRIEND

Sometimes your best workout buddy is right under your nose—or right under your feet. Dogs are a great excuse to get moving.

Dogs love bones, and you'll love your bones when you walk with your pup every day. Barbara Drinkwater, Ph.D., takes along a Frisbee to throw to her Border collie to exercise her arms and shoulders when they go for walks on her 20-acre farm.

If you aren't as lucky as Dr. Drinkwater and don't live in the country, you still can toss a ball or stick in the backyard or take the dog on a brisk stroll through the park.

Be mindful of rambunctious dogs, however, that can take you on a wild ride if they aren't trained to behave on a leash. You don't want to risk falling or tripping while trying to keep up with your four-footed friend. A good harness, a choke collar, or obedience lessons might be a wise investment if Fifi needs some remedial reminders to behave.

If you can't manage the upkeep of a dog but like the motivation, contact your local animal shelter, such as the Humane Society, where you can volunteer as a dog walker.

—Barbara Drinkwater, Ph.D., *is a research physiologist at Pacific Medical Center in Seattle.*

Strong
Bones
for Life

"*Bone health is a cumulative process. What you do every single day of your life has some bearing on what your risk of fractures is going to be.*"

—David J. Sartoris, M.D.,
professor of radiology and the director of bone densitometry, University of California, San Diego, School of Medicine

BE AN EARLY BIRD TO GET THE BONE

It's never too soon to understand and practice good bone health, beginning with nutrition, exercise, bone scans, and knowing risk factors.

The best time to build new bone and maximize bone health is during the first 3 decades of life. Until you reach the age of about 35, you build and store bone efficiently.

After that, bones begin to break down faster than new bone can be formed. In women, bone loss accelerates after menopause, when the ovaries stop producing estrogen, the hormone that protects against bone loss.

"We tend to focus on calcium, diet, and exercise requirements for the elderly—and we should—but their daughters and granddaughters will reap the greatest benefit from following this advice," says Michael A. Levine, M.D.

When you sit your daughter or niece down for the inevitable birds and the bees talk, consider adding another "B" to the list of topics—bones. It's true that it's never too late to stop bone loss, but you're certainly better off if you're early.

—Michael A. Levine, M.D., *is the director of pediatric endocrinology at the Johns Hopkins University School of Medicine in Baltimore.*

SUNBATHE FOR YOUR SKELETON

The only role you have to play in the unique biochemical process of getting vitamin D is to spend some time in the sun—and protect your skin from getting too much exposure.

It's a chain reaction. The sun's ultraviolet rays on your skin stimulate your body to produce vitamin D. Vitamin D enhances intestinal absorption of calcium. And as you probably know, calcium helps decrease bone loss.

Mornings and late afternoons, before 10:00 A.M. and after 2:00 P.M., are the best times to spend outdoors, because the sun's ultraviolet rays are least threatening to skin during those hours, says Tori Hudson, N.D.

Just don't sacrifice your skin for your skeleton. Wear sunscreen with a sun protection factor (SPF) of 15, a strength that blocks out some, but not all, of the sun's ultraviolet rays, says Dr. Hudson. Also, don't forget your UV-protecting sunglasses or a hat.

—Tori Hudson, N.D., *is professor at the National College of Naturopathic Medicine, the director of A Woman's Time in Portland, Oregon, and author of* Women's Encyclopedia of Natural Medicine.

FALL-PROOF YOUR HOME

Upturned carpeting and slippery floors
are just a few of the common household
hazards that could cause you to tumble.

Falls cause more than 90 percent of hip fractures, which can be disabling, says Chad Deal, M.D. That's why preventing falls is so important.

Danger zones around the house include loose rugs, protruding electrical cords, and a left-out pair of shoes. You need to develop an awareness of countless small or overlooked things that either get *in* the way or don't get *out* of the way.

What can you do? In short, if anything has the potential to move, nail (or glue or tape) it down. Secure any carpet edges that have come loose. Move cords against the wall and tape them down, if necessary. Apply nonskid backing to floor rugs, consider grab bars for the bathroom, and make sure that all steps and staircases—inside and outside of your home—have hand railings.

When everything is secured, tell your nephew he can't let his turtle run loose, and insist that your son not leave his baseball mitt on the steps. Safety is a convenient excuse to require your family to practice clutter control.

Also, make sure that you have proper lighting throughout the house. Night-lights are wise in case you need to get up in the middle of the night. You'll be able to see in case anyone forgot to put a pair of roller skates away.

—Chad Deal, M.D., *is the head of the center for osteoporosis and metabolic bone disease at the Cleveland Clinic.*

LOSE WEIGHT
WITHOUT LOSING BONES

*Taking off excess pounds can be the key
to a longer and healthier life for many
adults. But you do need to diet sensibly in
order to minimize or prevent bone loss.*

You shed more than fat and muscle when you lose weight—
you also lose bone, says Sue A. Shapses, Ph.D. As a rule
of thumb, you lose approximately 1 to 2 percent of your bone
mass for every 10 percent of weight loss, she says.

If you're overweight, don't let fear of bone loss deter you
from your weight-loss goals, says Dr. Shapses. But be certain
to shun fad diets, such as high-protein plans, or starvation
strategies, which could compromise your bones by keeping
you from getting all the nutrients you need.

Instead, choose a diet plan that emphasizes a variety of
healthy foods, including plenty of fruits and vegetables,
which have been linked with good bone density. Also, make
sure you're getting 1,500 milligrams of calcium and 600 IU
of vitamin D. If you're not getting enough of these nutrients
from the foods you eat, take supplements, says Dr. Shapses.

Be sure to combine any low-fat eating plan with weight-
bearing exercises, such as those described in Skeletal
Strength through Exercise on page 39. You'll not only burn
more calories but also help maintain bone mass by stimulating your skeleton with the stress of your impact—despite
the extra pounds you're taking off.

—Sue A. Shapses, Ph.D., *is associate professor of
nutritional sciences at Rutgers University in New Brunswick,
New Jersey.*

DON'T LET YOUR BONES FIZZLE OUT

*Those bubbly soft drinks can deplete
your bones of the calcium they need.
When you're thirsty, reach instead for
water, which promotes a more positive
nutrient balance.*

Soft drinks contain phosphoric acid, which leaches calcium from the bone, says Angela Stengler, N.D. Many varieties of soft drinks also contain caffeine and sugar, two more calcium-robbers.

Rather than reaching for the bubbly stuff, it's best to guzzle some water. Water clearly has many things going for it, including zero calories and fat.

Among the benefits, water lubricates joints, boosts energy, and guards against dehydration. It also helps the body maintain a proper balance of fluids, which in turn helps the bloodstream move nutrients (including bone-precious calcium) from one part of the body to another.

—Angela Stengler, N.D., *is a naturopathic physician in Oceanside, California, and coauthor of* Build Strong Bones: Prevent Osteoporosis and Enhance Bone Health Naturally.

HAVE AN
ALTERNATIVE BARBECUE

There are many activities you might associate with eating meat, like Fourth of July and Labor Day cookouts. But if you're trying to limit your animal protein consumption for healthier bones, get creative with the party cuisine.

The next time you fire up the grill, slap down a few veggie burgers instead of hamburgers. Add some great multigrain buns, some pickles, mayo, lettuce, and tomato, and voilà—the perfect burgers for the bone-savvy.

There are many types of vegetarian burgers available in health food stores and grocery stores, but try to find one that says it's for grilling, or one that's soy-based (looks like red meat), which holds together better and stays moister over flames than grain-based burgers.

For a gourmet alternative, grill some marinated, fresh vegetables such as eggplant, red bell peppers, summer squash, onions, and portobello mushrooms. You can always leave out the pork in your baked beans and make your chili vegetarian by substituting bulgur wheat for beef.

So what's all this beef with, well, beef? Red meat is the most protein-dense food. And too much protein can increase calcium loss in the urine and therefore boost your risk for osteoporosis, says Angela Stengler, N.D. Blame it on protein's high acid content. When protein breaks down, the body takes calcium from the bones to buffer the excess acid.

In general, safer sources of protein include fish, poultry, and legumes, says Dr. Stengler. These foods contain less protein, not to mention less saturated fat than red meat. If you enjoy the occasional steak or burger, limit yourself to one 6-ounce serving per week. Then be sure to add more calcium-rich foods to protein-dense meals.

So go ahead and make some homemade ice cream with your cookout companions, or put some cheese on that veggie burger!

—Angela Stengler, N.D., *is a naturopathic physician in Oceanside, California, and coauthor of* Build Strong Bones: Prevent Osteoporosis and Enhance Bone Health Naturally.

REJUVENATE WITHOUT CAFFEINE

Take a break from your usual coffee break by trying alternatives that don't leach precious nutrients from your bones.

You already know that coffee, tea, and other caffeinated beverages might make you feel more alert, but that wide-awake feeling comes at a price: Caffeine promotes the loss of calcium, magnesium, and other bone-building nutrients through the urine. The result is increased risk of fractures, reminds Mark Stengler, N.D.

A better alternative to coffee, tea, and other high-caffeine drinks is green tea, which has only one-fourth the caffeine of coffee and also has antioxidants that protect against heart disease and cancer, says Dr. Stengler. Better yet, get hooked on energy-enhancing herbal teas, such as peppermint or ginseng, he suggests.

The best way to beat an afternoon slump is by taking a walk around your building. If you can't get out, try lying on your back and swinging your legs up a wall. Having your feet suspended above your head brings more blood to your thyroid and head, rather than pooling it down in your feet. Accompany this wake-up pose with more rigorous stretches, and you'll feel alert—without the caffeine kickback that just makes you feel like you're needing more in a few hours.

If you're legitimately tired, maybe you should just give in to your fatigue and take a power nap. So long as you nap for less than a half-hour, and it's still the early part of the afternoon, sleep experts say you should feel refreshed.

—Mark Stengler, N.D., *is a naturopathic physician in Oceanside, California, and coauthor of* Build Strong Bones: Prevent Osteoporosis and Enhance Bone Health Naturally.

DON'T LET HEAVY METALS ROCK YOUR BONES

Those aluminum pots and pans in your kitchen might be cooking up some trouble for your bones.

High levels of toxic metals in the blood tend to deplete the body of bone-building essential minerals such as calcium, magnesium, and boron, says Irene Catania, N.D. "Aluminum is one mineral that could compete with necessary minerals in your body and could chelate or pull out calcium in the bones," she says.

When possible, avoid products containing aluminum. Rather than aluminum cookware, consider iron pans and glass pots.

Lesser-known sources of aluminum are most antiperspirants and other personal care products. Buy your antiperspirants at health food stores that sell products labeled aluminum-free. And when you have a choice, choose beverages in glass bottles over beverages in aluminum cans, says Dr. Catania. If you're using antacids, be sure to read the label first to rule out brands that contain aluminum.

—Irene Catania, N.D., *is a naturopathic physician in Ho-Ho-Kus, New Jersey.*

DON'T CELEBRATE WITH SUGAR

Treating yourself to too many sugary foods is not sweet to your bones.

Some of us never outgrew the childhood habit of rewarding ourselves with candy. We earn a good commission at work, so we pick up a box of glazed doughnuts. We finally stand up to a bully coworker, and we devour a candy bar. When we're miserable, we console ourselves with sugar foods, too.

Cookies, candy, ice cream, and other treats might be all right for an occasional decadent indulgence. But a steady supply of sugar could jeopardize your bones because calcium is lost in the urine after eating sugary foods, says Mark Stengler, N.D.

Another reason to forgo the dessert habit is that we already get a steady supply of sugar in our daily diet from staples such as pasta, bread, and fruit juice. In fact, sugar is found in virtually every processed food, says Dr. Stengler. That's a lot of calcium loss.

Instead, reward yourself with something that's more deeply satisfying than a box of caramel corn and a soda, like a full-body massage or a facial on your lunch break. Or when you have a celebratory meal, top it off with a moonlight walk in a local park rather than cake.

You could always use your candy money for a dynamite new pair of earrings. They will last longer than gobbling down a nougat bar *and* are fat-free.

—Mark Stengler, N.D., *is a naturopathic physician in Oceanside, California, and coauthor of* Build Strong Bones: Prevent Osteoporosis and Enhance Bone Health Naturally.

NIX THE NICOTINE

Need another reason to stub out those butts for good? A woman who is a lifelong smoker doubles her risk of osteoporotic fractures.

Smoking harms bones in several ways. For starters, it causes a more rapid metabolism of estrogen, and bone breaks down faster when estrogen levels drop.

"People who are lifelong smokers, especially people who start smoking in their adolescent years, don't ever achieve the peak bone mass that nonsmokers do," says Chad Deal, M.D.

Smokers also tend to be more frail than nonsmokers because cigarette smoke affects muscle health and strength, says Dr. Deal. That means people who smoke are more likely to experience accidental falls. To make matters worse, smokers generally don't exercise as much as nonsmokers, and people who are sedentary have a greater risk for bone loss than people who are active, he adds.

If you'd like to quit but aren't sure how to do it, contact the American Lung Association at 1740 Broadway, New York, NY 10019-4371, or look in the newspaper for your local office.

—Chad Deal, M.D., *is the head of the center for osteoporosis and metabolic bone disease at the Cleveland Clinic.*

SHAKE SALT OUT OF YOUR KITCHEN

You usually don't know how much sodium you're consuming when you're eating ready-made food, but you can assume it's excessive. Cooking at home is your opportunity to flavor food with other, more interesting options.

Most Americans eat 3,000 to 6,000 milligrams of salt daily. There's no minimum requirement, but this is far more than we need to fulfill salt's main function of maintaining proper body fluids. A high salt intake is considered a risk factor for osteoporosis because it causes calcium loss through the kidneys, says Michael A. Levine, M.D.

So throw salt over your shoulder, not in a pot of your homemade stew. With any luck, you'll keep your calcium levels up by cooking at home rather than being fed by a salt-laced processed food industry.

Explore the many flavoring agents other than those same old white granules. Chances are, your dishes will be so enticing that you won't miss salt. In fact, if you gradually decrease the amount of salt in your diet, your taste for it wanes, says Dr. Levine.

Here are some ways to reduce your salt intake without cutting back on flavor.

- Sprinkle tasty nutritional yeast and Cajun spices over home-popped popcorn sprayed with olive oil.
- Squeeze lemon juice on steamed vegetables and broiled fish.
- Experiment with salsa or hot sauce on staples such as eggs, rice, and potatoes.
- Season soups with salt-free garlic and herb seasoning as well as with flavored vinegars.
- Add 1 heaping teaspoon of salt-free Italian seasoning blend to the boiling water when you make pasta.
- Switch to reduced-sodium table salt.
- Slather your corn on the cob with olive oil and garlic powder or unsalted butter.
- Rather than salt-drenched soy sauce on Asian food, substitute similar-tasting liquid aminos, which are derived from vegetable proteins with minimal naturally occurring sodium. Liquid aminos, such as the Bragg brand, are available at natural food markets.

—Michael A. Levine, M.D., *is the director of pediatric endocrinology at the Johns Hopkins University School of Medicine in Baltimore.*

BE HIP ABOUT BENDING

*Bending from the hips saves your spine
in a lot of everyday situations.*

Typical daily chores, like unloading the dishwasher or making the bed, often require you to bend over. It feels natural to bend from the waist at these times, but doing so can increase the risk of spinal fractures for a person with a weakened skeleton, says Margie Bissinger, P.T.

"It's important that you bend from the hips and not from the waist," she says. The hips are located deep in the folds where your legs join your trunk, she says. Think of your body as being divided into an upper and a lower half, with the hips being the dividing line. This is where the bending motion should take place.

In order to bend from your hips, your trunk needs to be straight. So put your hands on your stomach and back before bending. Leading with your head and chest, bend forward with the movement occurring at the hips and knees, says Bissinger. Your lower back should keep its natural curve.

Once you've practiced this better way of bending, be sure to implement it in your daily routine. It's also a good way to avoid discomfort (and even potential injury) when you get into and out of a chair, says Bissinger.

—Margie Bissinger, P.T., *is a licensed physical therapist in Parsippany, New Jersey, director of Workfit Consultants, and author of* Osteoporosis: An Exercise Guide.

THINK BEFORE YOU LIFT

A back that might already be compromised by weak bones shouldn't have the extra burden of careless lifting. Respect your spine by limiting your load and using the best form.

It's always tempting to grab all the groceries from the car to avoid a second trip. After all, who likes the extra trouble when the ice cream is melting, the cats are nosing through your bags, and you just want to unload and unwind? But even so, you need to lift less and use the smartest techniques to avoid injury, says Mary Pullig Schatz, M.D.

Here's the smart-lifting style Dr. Schatz recommends.

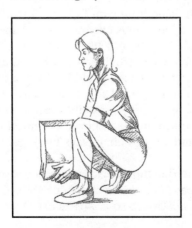

Position yourself near the grocery bag or anything else you want to lift. Place your feet about shoulder-width apart. Keep one leg slightly forward and alongside the bag. Now, lower yourself by bending your knees. Be sure to keep your back straight and upright.

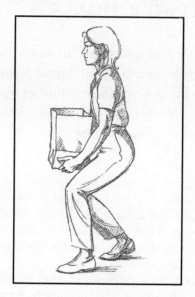

Hug the bag to your body and stand up by pushing down strongly with both feet as you straighten your legs.

Of course, groceries aren't the only weighty things we encounter from day to day. Even lifting small children can put a serious strain on the back. To safely lift a child, try the following: Lower one knee to the floor. Ask the toddler to put her arms around you, hold her close to your body, then lift up. Keep your abdominal muscles contracted as you lift for added support.

—Mary Pullig Schatz, M.D., is a yoga instructor in Nashville and author of Back Care Basics.

RELAX FOR
STRONGER BONES

A nightly foot massage can soothe tension while keeping your bones strong. What's the connection? Rubbing out stress is important for bone health as well as emotional health.

There's actually a biochemical link between stress and bone health, says Irene Catania, N.D. The adrenal glands produce DHEA, a precursor for female hormones such as estrogen. When tension inhibits the adrenal glands, the body produces less DHEA and, therefore, a lower volume of bone-protecting hormones.

Stress can harm your bones in other ways, too, says Dr. Catania. Stress produces cell-damaging free radicals, which are unstable molecules that pilfer electrons from your body's healthy molecules to balance themselves. Free radicals can contribute to an acid pH imbalance in the body. In an effort to buffer the blood and balance the pH, calcium gets pulled out of body tissues, including bones.

One quick and easy way to alleviate stress is a 5-minute foot massage. According to the traditions of reflexology, the bottom of the foot correlates to every organ and gland in the body. "By rubbing the bottom of your foot, you're sending a message to every place in the body to relax and calm down," Dr. Catania says.

Select an herbal oil with a calming scent, such as lavender. Before bedtime, massage the entire sole of the foot, including the toes. Pay special attention to any tender spots, as these often indicate areas that need more massage, says Dr. Catania. Be thorough, but don't overdo it.

—Irene Catania, N.D., *is a naturopathic physician in Ho-Ho-Kus, New Jersey.*

KNOW THE SIGNS OF MENOPAUSE

Hot flashes, night sweats, heart palpitations, and mood swings signal more than the onset of menopause. They're also telling you that your bones need special attention.

Gradual bone loss is an inevitable part of aging, says Tori Hudson, N.D. But women lose bone most rapidly during the first few years of menopause, as estrogen and other potentially bone-protecting hormones such as progesterone and DHEA decline.

Other menopausal symptoms include insomnia, irregular menstrual bleeding, vaginal dryness, and feelings of depression and anxiety. If you already take steps to protect your bones, then you're doing great. Keep up the good work. But if you haven't been as kind to your bones as you should have been, then consider early menopause as the "last call" for your bones.

Now is the time to pay serious attention to exercise, diet, stress, and other lifestyle issues in an effort to help offset the rapid bone loss that tends to accompany menopause, says Dr. Hudson.

—Tori Hudson, N.D., *is professor at the National College of Naturopathic Medicine, director of A Woman's Time in Portland, Oregon, and author of* Women's Encyclopedia of Natural Medicine.

CIRCULATE. . . DON'T CIRCLE!

Even if you eat well, your bones might be starved for calcium. Good circulation is needed in order to process those nutrients, and you can get it with an active lifestyle.

Think of all the times you circled the parking lot at work or the grocery store in search of the primo spot to park your car. You know—the one that's closest to your destination. Well, it's time to reconsider that strategy. Parking your car at a reasonable distance from the door gives you a chance to get moving and therefore improve your circulation.

Proper circulation is important for bone health because it brings nutrients such as calcium to cells and removes toxins from the blood, explains Irene Catania, N.D. "Circulation is an indirect but necessary component of good bone health," she says. "If you get enough calcium and other bone-building minerals in your diet but your circulation is sluggish, then you might not have the best nutritional status."

The bottom line: Fight a sedentary lifestyle. Don't rely on elevators, golf carts, electric mixers, and those prized parking spots. . . unless it's pouring rain.

—Irene Catania, N.D., *is a naturopathic physician in Ho-Ho-Kus, New Jersey.*

TRY AN ALTERNATIVE TO SEDATIVES

Watch your step when taking sedatives. A drugged-up, groggy state can set you up for debilitating or fatal fractures.

People who take certain sedatives sometimes get up in the middle of the night. They are drowsy and lose their footing, explains Chad Deal, M.D. This is something to take very seriously, because falls can cause hip fractures, which can be deadly, he says.

Valium, Elavil, and other medications with a long-acting sedative effect can trip you up the most. If you need some help falling asleep, try using shorter-acting sedatives such as Benadryl. An herbal alternative is to drink tea brewed from chamomile, oatstraw, and catnip. You could also try an extract of the herb kava kava to calm you before sleep. Follow the package directions. These natural sedatives won't leave you with a groggy feeling.

Another safe snoozing option is to develop a calming bedtime ritual, like taking a warm bath, listening to soothing music, or reading for pleasure before turning off the lights.

Also, avoid caffeinated products. Consumed as early as 2:00 P.M., they can disturb your nightly sleep, warns Dr. Deal.

Be aware that diuretics (medications that cause you to lose water) can also lead to falls. These medications cause a drop in blood pressure when you stand up, making you lightheaded and unsteady.

—Chad Deal, M.D., *is the head of the center for osteoporosis and metabolic bone disease at the Cleveland Clinic.*

Living Well with Brittle Bones

"Living out an active, healthy lifestyle will make you feel better and can even help you maintain or increase what bone density you have."

—Margie Bissinger, P.T.,
licensed physical therapist in Parsippany, New Jersey, director of Workfit Consultants, and author of Osteoporosis: An Exercise Guide

DON'T LET YOUR PET TRIP YOU UP

Because falls can more easily lead to fractures when you have brittle bones, you need to be aware of where your furry friends are lurking. Try this charming cat or dog alert system.

Cats and dogs are only looking for affection when they cling near to your ankles. But if you have osteoporosis, their "affection" can be a real and present danger to you, especially if your balance isn't the greatest, says Theresa D. Galsworthy, R.N.

A simple way to make your little buddy more noticeable around the house is to tie a bell on his collar. That way, every time he comes by, you'll hear the tinkling and be able to look out below. Although you'll still need to be observant of pets sleeping or sitting on the floor, says Galsworthy, at least the moving ones will make their presence known.

Remember, also, that some pets can get pretty rambunctious around feeding times, so hold on to something like a banister or a stable table ledge when you're setting down your pet's food dish.

—Theresa D. Galsworthy, R.N., *is the cofounder and director of the osteoporosis prevention center at the Hospital for Special Surgery in New York City.*

GARDENERS: GO FOUR-WHEELIN'

Don't risk a fracture when you're pushing leaves and mulch around your yard with a precarious wheelbarrow. Switch to a cart that's smart for your safety.

Tending your flowers and vegetables is actually a healthy hobby for developing stronger bones. Gardening incorporates walking, lifting, and pulling for a bit of weight-bearing activity. All that said, backyard farmers be forewarned: If you have brittle bones, watch out for the not-so-obvious hazards that can make you fall. A big garden gamble is the wheelbarrow.

Vincent Schaller, M.D., who sees many people with osteoporosis in his private practice, warns that wheelbarrows by nature are wobbly and can easily cause a person to slip and fall.

He suggests that gardeners with osteoporosis use one of the four-wheeled carts available in many stores that sell garden supplies. These carts are more stable and also have larger wheels, like a bicycle, which makes them easier to maneuver.

Besides dumping the old wheelbarrow, Dr. Schaller reminds you to make the ground in your yard and gardens more level by incorporating things like flat stepping stones and wider vegetable beds. Watch out for rabbit holes, slippery mud, and other dangerous footing, too.

—Vincent Schaller, M.D., *is a family physician and partner at Dover Family Physicians in Dover, Delaware.*

GET YOUR HIPS A CRASH HELMET

The link between decreased bone mass and increased hip fractures is something to take seriously. If your bones are very brittle, wearing a hip protector can bring you safety and security.

Once a hip is broken, nearly half of the people with osteoporosis sustain serious enough injuries to lose their mobility. Hip protectors can reduce the chance of fracture by dispersing and absorbing the impact of a fall across the soft tissue in your hip area, so your bone doesn't take the full jolt of a fall, says Jes Bruun Lauritzen, M.D.

There are various hip padding systems, from one that acts like a mini airbag to one that resembles a soft horseshoe around your hips. The most promising design is a crash-helmet-type hip protector that uses two stiff polypropylene shells sewn into bicycle-style shorts and is worn discreetly under clothes.

In a study at the University of Copenhagen's medical school hospital, seniors who wore this type of hip protector had 50 percent fewer fractures than those who didn't have protection. A Swedish repeat study also found a 50 percent reduction with women who were even more frail.

Hip protectors can be purchased through Safehip, 601 Park East Drive, Woonsocket, RI 02895.

—Jes Bruun Lauritzen, M.D., *is associate professor in orthopedic surgery at the University of Copenhagen's Hvidovre Hospital in Denmark.*

PRACTICE HEALTHY HOUSEKEEPING

If you want to avoid pain and potential injury to your spine, you need to use the right technique for everyday chores.

Somebody has to do all those little tasks to keep a home orderly and sanitary. If that somebody is you, be sure to avoid hurting your brittle spine. Margie Bissinger, P.T., offers the golden rules of spine-safe housework. They can be applied to vaccuming, mopping, and even raking.

- Don't bend from the waist. Instead, bend from the hips and knees.
- Don't twist and bend simultaneously. This puts excessive stress on the spine, predisposing it to injury.
- It's always better to push rather than pull an object, if you have a choice. Pushing is much easier for your back, because you utilize your leg muscles to do most of the work. It's also a more stable position.
- When moving the vacuum, mop, or rake back and forth, place one leg in front of the other, knees bent, and rock from foot to foot. All the while, you should keep your spine in a lengthened position, instead of hunched over.
- If you're moving a mop or a rake sideways, be sure to stand with your legs spread shoulder-width apart. Then rock sideways from leg to leg. If you twist your spine instead, you'll risk injury.

—Margie Bissinger, P.T., *is a licensed physical therapist in Parsippany, New Jersey, director of Workfit Consultants, and author of* Osteoporosis: An Exercise Guide.

CHOOSE A BONE-SAFE VEHICLE

Whether you're shopping for a new vehicle or just trying to choose between family cars, don't get stuck with one that's bad to the bone.

Getting into and out of a car is a big deal to someone with osteoporosis. One false move can lay you flat on the ground with a fractured hip.

Vincent Schaller, M.D., says that drivers need to think carefully about getting enough clearance when they get into and out of the front seat. "People fall because they can't get good footing when they don't have a lot of room to maneuver into or out of the seat," he says.

Minivans and small trucks provide a good deal of room for you to swing yourself around and boost yourself out of the vehicle. Two-door model cars tend to offer more clearance than four-door ones. Because every model is different, carefully test out the door-opening space of a car before you commit to buying it.

Of course, four doors make getting in and out of a vehicle easier for people in the *back* seat—something to keep in mind when you have passengers with osteoporosis, says Dr. Schaller.

Parking on paved, level ground will help you reduce the risk of falls, regardless of what car you're in at the time, Dr. Schaller adds.

—Vincent Schaller, M.D., *is a family physician and partner at Dover Family Physicians in Dover, Delaware.*

COUGH AND SNEEZE WITH EASE

Don't let the sudden force of a sneeze or cough put your spine in jeopardy. Brace your back when you feel one coming on.

For a person with a weakened skeleton, a cough or sneeze is, well, nothing to sneeze at.

"The sudden force of a cough or sneeze can cause your spine to bend forward suddenly, which can lead to injuries of the spine and vertebral fractures," explains Margie Bissinger, P.T.

Bissinger says it's very important to stabilize your back in anticipation of a cough or sneeze. You can place one hand on the small of your lower back to help you stand erect during the sneeze. Or you can bend your knees and hips, keeping your back lengthened (instead of hunched over), and place one hand on your thigh. This will help stabilize your back and keep it in alignment when you cough or sneeze, says Bissinger.

Practice these techniques so that you're ready for action the next time you feel as if you're going to sneeze or cough. After a while, it should become second nature for you to position yourself this way.

—Margie Bissinger, P.T., *is a licensed physical therapist in Parsippany, New Jersey, director of Workfit Consultants, and author of* Osteoporosis: An Exercise Guide.

WEAR RUNNING SHOES, EVEN IF YOU NEVER RUN

Whether you're at work or at play, wearing running shoes can help reduce discomfort and keep you free from injury.

According to James S. Adleberg, D.P.M., P.A., you should wear a well-cushioned, supportive shoe with good shock absorption every day. This will help protect your lower back from the relentless pounding it takes as you go about your day.

"I normally recommend a running shoe variety to my patients," says Dr. Adleberg. Running shoes are lightweight, and they tend to be more supportive and a lot more shock absorbing than walking shoes. And unlike high heels and other flimsily constructed shoes, running sneakers might just help you maintain better footing, thus reducing your chance of falling.

To find a good pair of running shoes, go to a reputable athletic shoe store. Remember that your shoe should feel comfortable and not feel that it needs to be broken in. When you walk around, there should be no slippage in the heel, and there should be enough room in the toes so they don't feel crowded.

—James S. Adleberg, D.P.M., P.A., *is an attending physician at Mercy Medical Center in Baltimore and a podiatrist in private practice.*

REPLACE YOUR SHOES

Just because the shoe still fits doesn't mean it still provides the necessary support and shock absorption your bones need.

You love those snazzy sneakers you bought for walking last year, and you wear them almost every day. But no matter how nice they appear, it's probably time to move on.

"I recommend that if somebody is wearing shoes for any type of exercise, including walking, they should replace their shoes at least once a year—especially if they have osteoporosis," says James S. Adleberg, D.P.M., P.A. The materials in the midsole (inside the bottom part of the shoe) wear out after a while. Then they can no longer offer you enough shock absorption and support.

"It's really important for shoe gear to be in good shape because your feet hit the ground first, and part of their job is to help limit shock from traveling up your legs and into your spinal column," says Dr. Adleberg.

—James S. Adleberg, D.P.M., P.A., *is an attending physician at Mercy Medical Center in Baltimore and a podiatrist in private practice.*

CARRY-ON YOUR COMFORT

Take a load off your back when you travel by making good use of your luggage. Your bag can do double duty as a posture-correcting footrest.

If you have brittle bones, make travel by plane, train, or bus a bit easier on your lower back by stowing your carry-on luggage under the seat in front of you, instead of in an overhead compartment. It's not just that slugging your bag overhead can harm your spine, but you can also assume the safest and most comfortable posture by using a bag on the floor as a footrest.

Allan Magaziner, D.O., says that keeping your feet 4 to 6 inches above ground will keep the top part of your legs parallel to the floor, which can help correct an undesirable curvature of your lower back while you sit. Your footrest will also train you to sit in a position that can strengthen a weakened back over time.

—Allan Magaziner, D.O., *is the founder and director of the Magaziner Center for Wellness and Anti-Aging Medicine in Cherry Hill, New Jersey.*

TAKE A STEP
IN THE RIGHT DIRECTION

If you have hunched-over posture from osteoporosis, standing for long periods of time can make your poor posture worse, not to mention cause a tight, achy back, neck, and shoulders. A simple step stool can improve your stance.

You might think of a step stool as being a tool of the trade for a librarian or inventory clerk who needs to reach high places. But even if you're a cashier or traffic director who stays in the same place all day, it can be an invaluable tool, particularly if your spine is weakened from osteoporosis.

"Put one foot up on the bottom step of a step stool, alternating which leg is raised periodically," instructs Russell E. Windsor, M.D. "This changes the curvature of your spine, so your stance is more correct and comfortable."

If you don't have a step stool handy, you can try a footrest. Although it won't give you as much beneficial curvature as a taller stool, footrests are inexpensive and still effective, he says.

—Russell E. Windsor, M.D., *is professor of orthopedic surgery at the Weill Medical College of Cornell University and a surgeon and physician at the Hospital for Special Surgery, both in New York City.*

Throw In the Towel
for Auto Travel

*Spending too much time in a car can
really cause a lot of back discomfort,
especially if you have osteoporosis. A
simple rolled-up towel behind your back
will keep you motoring in comfort.*

If you have a weakened skeleton, sitting in a car for a long time can be more than uncomfortable. It can put excessive pressure on your spine.

"Really, the best thing to do during long drives is to get out of the car every couple of hours and stand up or walk around," says Robert Uebele, P.T. But he acknowledges that this isn't always an option when you're stuck in traffic or need to make fast tracks. In those instances, a rolled-up towel might be your best option for finding relief.

Roll up a regular bath towel and place it, horizontally, behind the lumbar area of your spine (that's the lower back, where the curve is). Then sit against the backrest of your seat. This makes you sit straighter. The result: less pressure on the spine, and less pain.

A rolled-up towel works on office chairs and airplane seats, too. It's cheaper and more adjustable than commercial back-support pillows—not to mention easier to wash, Uebele says.

—Robert Uebele, P.T., *is the clinical coordinator for the rehabilitation unit at Bayhealth Medical Center in Milford, Delaware.*

CONSIDER MAGNETS FOR RELIEF

Try magnets if you're attracted to their potential to relieve osteoporosis-related pain.

Therapeutic magnets are worn in braces around the back, knees, ankles, and wrists. Some people sleep on mattress pads full of them. The medical community might be skeptical, but people who have worn them over an area of chronic pain claim relief where nothing else has worked.

"Magnets really are remarkable for pain," says Janet Zand, O.M.D., L.Ac., a doctor of Oriental medicine and naturopathic physician who treats osteoporosis patients with magnets. Dr. Zand directs her osteoporosis patients to place magnets on the area of pain as well as on acupuncture points.

Magnets are safe to try because they don't usually have any dangerous side effects, says Dr. Zand. The only warning she has is that, on rare occasions, people can become overstimulated by the magnet. Taking the magnets off before bedtime should prevent overstimulation.

If you don't get them from your alternative practitioner, you'll receive directions as part of a kit when you purchase magnets at sporting goods stores, at health food stores, through mail order, or from private distributors. Not all magnets are the same strength or suit your needs. Prices vary greatly, depending on the size and strength of the magnets. Small ones run about $25, and magnet-filled mattress pads sell for several hundred dollars.

Your best bet is to purchase products with a money-back guarantee if you're not satisfied. Also, buy a magnet that is at least 400 gauss in strength.

—Janet Zand, O.M.D., L.Ac., *is the chairperson and formulator for Zand Herbal in Boulder, Colorado, and author of* Smart Medicine for Healthier Living, *with a private medical practice in Austin, Texas, and Santa Monica, California.*

POSITION YOURSELF FOR PLEASURE

Sex should never become uncomfortable due to brittle bones. Experiment with ways to maintain maximum pleasure during lovemaking.

I f you have pain during sex, ask your partner to work with you to find specific positions or techniques that will eliminate the pain. "You need to talk about ways to keep things comfortable, thus enjoyable, for both of you," says Theresa D. Galsworthy, R.N., who has worked with thousands of osteoporosis patients.

You'll find that there are many creative ways to avoid problems. For example, being on top or in a side-to-side position might generally be easier on a woman's weakened skeleton, she says.

If you're underneath, it might be more comfortable if your partner supports his weight on his arms. That way, you don't have added pressure on your spine or hips from your lover's body.

Placing a pillow under the lumbar area of the spine (where the lower back arches) while you're lying on your back might also help. You also might want to initiate sitting on a chair or table to take excess body weight off your weakened spine.

If you're experiencing spinal or hip pain during sex, don't hesitate to discuss this with your doctor, who might be able to tell you about specific positions or techniques that can help your individual situation.

—Theresa D. Galsworthy, R.N., *is the cofounder and director of the osteoporosis prevention center at the Hospital for Special Surgery in New York City.*

MAKE FASHION FUNCTION FOR YOU

You don't have to choose between fashion and comfort just because osteoporosis has caused changes in your figure.

If you've developed the curving back and shoulders, loss of height, and thickening waistline that are characteristic of compression fractures of the spine, you can't pull out your favorite old standards in the closet and flaunt them the same way. It's also harder to pick what you want off the rack and expect it to fit right. Instead, you might find jackets and blouses pulling across your back and shoulders, gaping collars, and skirts that don't hang properly.

Nonetheless, brittle bones don't change the fact that you want to look good, says Janna C. Kimel, president of Accessible Threads, a custom clothing and alterations company for people with special needs. Whether you're altering existing pieces or shopping for new clothing, there are lots of tricks to hide the effects of osteoporosis, she says.

When one hip is higher than the other, it's best to even out the skirt or pants by altering them at the waistline, not at the hem. This will create an even-looking hem on the bottom, she says. For an easier dressing modification, she recommends replacing zippers and buttons with Velcro.

If you prefer to leave the sewing to the experts, expect to pay about $25 an hour for alterations, and $100 for custom-made clothes where you can pick out your own favorite fabrics and styles.

If you prefer to forgo the tailor, consider this shopping advice.

• Long scarves or shawls give a longer profile from the back, while they also highlight the face and draw eyes away from the shoulder area. A shorter scarf in bold, bright patterns can fill a gaping collar or neckline with flair.

• Wear a backpack rather than a purse to distribute your weight evenly.

• Shoulder pads can compensate for sloping shoulders.

• Choose tops with cowl, rounded, or slight V necklines as well as dropped or dolman sleeves.

• Find pants with elasticized waistlines.

• The best shirts are those that are slightly longer in the back.

—Janna C. Kimel *is the president and founder of Accessible Threads in Evanston, Illinois.*

SEEK EMOTIONAL SUPPORT

When your skeleton is weak, your spirit might need some bolstering, too. A community of people with osteoporosis can help you stand tall, while keeping you motivated and informed.

No one should feel that it's necessary to suffer alone with osteoporosis, says Margie Bissinger, P.T. A support group can answer questions and talk you through some tough emotional times as well as keep you focused on doing what's best for your bones.

To locate an osteoporosis support group, look in your local paper, call area hospitals, or contact the National Osteoporosis Foundation, which can help you find or even start one in your area. Write to Building Strength Together, 515 North State Street, Chicago, IL 60610 or e-mail NOF's manager of support group services at supgroup@nof.org.

Don't discount the Internet as a tool to meet your needs if attending a meeting is physically uncomfortable or impossible for you. You'll discover diet advice, exercise information, medication discussions, and cutting-edge research as well as opportunities to connect personally with people in chat rooms.

At the very least, consider subscribing to a magazine or newsletter that will keep you informed of current issues surrounding osteoporosis. Then, in the privacy of your own home, you can read other people's personal accounts of coping with their physical and emotional changes.

—Margie Bissinger, P.T., *is a licensed physical therapist in Parsippany, New Jersey, director of Workfit Consultants, and author of* Osteoporosis: An Exercise Guide.

Alternative Options

Because holistic healers will guide you to stay in a state of overall wellness, being under their care can prevent you from ever developing avoidable risk factors, such as high stress, smoking, and unhealthy dieting. Should you approach roadblocks that keep you from living your most bone-healthy lifestyle, alternative practitioners will draw on vast resources to help, using an array of cultures and philosophies.

You might be given, for example, meditations to motivate you to exercise, herbs to help you quit smoking, or acupuncture to overcome a food allergy that might prevent your intake of calcium-rich dairy foods.

For actual treatment of osteoporosis, you will find that the various holistic healers will offer solutions targeted at what they know about the uniqueness of your mind, body, and spirit. In other words, you will be offered alternative options that are more personalized than a conventional doctor's general dietary and lifestyle plans, and more natural than prescription medications.

For all stages of the disease, alternative practitioners have a wealth of resources to help you cope with special problems, such as bodywork to alleviate pain, herbs that can help bone recover from fracture, and water therapy to improve your mobility.

Many of these health professionals work in tandem with each other and with traditional medical doctors to give you a best-of-all-worlds approach. For example, the promising pharmaceutical drug prescribed by your physician might be enhanced by the advanced dietary advice that alternative doctors such as naturopaths and Ayurvedic practitioners can offer.

Use this guide as a resource to select a healer or build a team of healers who have the training you need to aggressively halt or even reverse bone loss.

Ayurvedic Medicine Specialists

Practitioners of Ayurveda, a 5,000-year-old healing system originating in India, consider osteoporosis to be an imbalance of the *vata* form of energy—one of the three principal energies or facets of one's being. The goal of Ayurvedic medicine is to balance the body's three principal energies so they can work together in harmony, since disease results from an imbalance among them.

To restore the balance of vata energy and thereby enhance the preservation and creation of strong bone, Ayurvedic doctors recommend dietary modifications, herbal and homeopathic remedies, and exercise that includes breathing techniques, yoga postures, daily walks, and underwater exercise.

Food is very much medicine for osteoporotic bones. If you are being treated by an Ayurvedic doctor for osteoporosis, expect to eat soy products, soaked almonds, white sesame seeds, yogurt, and aloe—and to take them in specific amounts at specific times of the day.

Central to the Ayurvedic approach is a keen focus on proper digestion, which is essential for enabling bones to utilize vital nutrients. Therefore, food combinations are carefully selected not only for their nutrients but also to enhance the vitamin and mineral uptake in the body.

For more information on Ayurveda, write to The Ayurvedic Institute at 11311 Menaul, NE, Albuquerque, NM 87112.

Feldenkrais Practitioners

People with osteoporosis often develop cramped and out-of-balance movements to accommodate for pain and injuries. Over time, the entire body will begin to feel the strain of poor posture, such as rounded-over shoulders and a slumping back. Using their system of retraining the nervous system, Feldenkrais practitioners help a person with osteoporosis make subtle shifts to bring the neck and spine back into alignment.

For a body that is deformed, they will teach more comfortable ways of standing, sitting, and walking to avoid pain and increase range of motion. For those with soft bones, Feldenkrais practitioners can help establish more stabilizing movements for avoiding injuries.

Trained in neurology, physiology, and psychology, a practitioner uses two basic techniques: The first, known as *functional integration*, involves one-on-one sessions on a padded table. In the first session the practitioner will conduct a "body scan" to feel for areas of tension and pain. Then she will gently guide your limbs through a series of custom-tailored movements to essentially train your brain and body to execute healthier motions.

The second technique is a series of group or private *awareness through movement* classes, in which voice cues are given to execute small gestures like bending, reaching, and leaning. At this time your instructor will offer suggestions regarding how you can move better.

According to Bonnie Kissam, a Feldenkrais practitioner in Hartford, Connecticut, you can feel the benefits after committing to a series of 8 to 10 sessions. But don't stop there—improving your movement and posture is an ongoing process.

An authorized Feldenkrais practitioner has completed 800 to 900 hours of study over a 4-year period in an approved Feldenkrais Guild Training Program. To locate an instructor or receive more information, contact the

Feldenkrais Guild of North America at 3611 Southwest Hood Avenue, Suite 100, Portland, OR 97201.

Herbalists

Health care professionals who specialize in herbal remedies have a variety of specific botanical medicines they use for women at risk for, or suffering from, osteoporosis. Tinctures, teas, and dried herb-filled capsules might be prescribed in different strengths for the individual needs of each person.

For osteoporosis prevention, herbal formulas might include plants that produce estrogen-like effects, such as dong quai, unicorn root, black cohosh, fennel, and licorice.

A variety of herbs might be prescribed that foster efficient digestion so that all the trace minerals and elements important to bone reach their targets, says Michael Moore, an herbalist who directs the Southwest School of Botanical Medicine in Bisbee, Arizona.

Moore teaches people to make fresh teas from such sources as dandelions, red clover, and alfalfa. He says these teas help calcium bypass the intestines, so it cannot be excreted before it reaches your bones.

During any phase of osteoporosis, herbalists will look to the earth for natural solutions to assist you in making better lifestyle choices. An herbalist can create a tincture for you to steadily and healthfully gain weight in order to strengthen your skeleton. Seek an herbalist for a formula to help with smoking cessation, or to reduce depression before it can interfere with your hormones (and, eventually, with your bone density). Herbalists even offer botanical medicine for osteoporosis-related pain, and solutions to insomnia that won't make you so groggy that you might fall and risk fracture.

To find a qualified herbalist in your area, contact the American Herbalists Guild at P. O. Box 70, Roosevelt, UT 84066.

Naturopathic Medicine

Being under the care of a licensed naturopathic physician is like having a doctor who has taken traditional medical school courses, yet is also trained in homeopathy, therapeutic nutrition, hydrotherapy, botanical medicine, spinal manipulation, and other alternative therapeutic modalities.

To treat you for osteoporosis, he mostly likely will offer sophisticated advice on vitamins, minerals, amino acids, and hormones as well as the quality of your digestion. He will also question environmental factors that could influence the way you utilize your nutrients.

Whereas hormone-replacement therapy (HRT) is prevalent in conventional care, naturopathic doctors generally agree that the risks of HRT outweigh the benefits. Many N.D.'s prefer to prescribe plant-based supplements that have estrogen-like effects, however. The main object of HRT is to inhibit bone loss and enhance formation of new bone.

Lyn Patrick, N.D., of Tucson recommends ipriflavone as a natural bone preserver. She also counsels her patients to protect themselves from osteoporosis by taking what she considers the most bioavailable form of calcium as well as trace minerals, including manganese, boron, zinc, copper, silicon, and hydroxy apatite.

Naturopathic doctors might stress whole foods, vegetarian diets for bone health, and a physically active lifestyle that includes strength and resistance training.

Seek out a member of The American Association of Naturopathic Physicians (AANP) to be sure a naturopath has had the proper in-depth training. For a directory of members, contact the AANP at 601 Valley Street, Suite 105, Seattle, WA 98109.

Traditional Oriental Medicine

According to traditional Chinese medicine, the kidneys rule the bones. Therefore, hand pressure, in the form of acupressure, or fine needles, in the form of acupuncture, are used to stimulate the flow of energy to the kidneys and digestive system.

In noneastern world terms, acupuncture (stimulation with fine needles) is helpful in maintaining hormone levels needed for building bone density, says JoAnn (Hickey) Tall, O.M.D., L.Ac., president of the Santa Barbara College of Oriental Medicine in California. In advanced stages of the disease, acupressure or acupuncture is recommended for relieving osteoporosis-related pain.

Of course, acupuncture doesn't work in a vacuum, but rather it's part of the whole mosaic of Oriental medicine, where the basis of health is considered to be the balance of life-giving energy, known as qi. Treatment for disease, including osteoporosis, involves restoring the energies within your body that have gotten out of sync or out of balance.

Other methods to restore balance include breathing exercises, meditation and visualization, herbs, and exercise. The gentle martial art of tai chi is highly recommended, because it enhances a person's energy forces while stimulating bone to regenerate. Dr. Tall also encourages people to lift light weights twice a week.

For information on locating Oriental medicine physicians, acupressurists, and acupuncturists, contact the American Association of Oriental Medicine (AAOM) at 433 Front Street, Catasauqua, PA 18032.

Yoga Masters

Properly taught by a well-trained instructor, yoga can be an excellent method to improve posture and enhance agility and body alignment, while also strengthening the spine—all key to the treatment of osteoporosis. And despite the gentle movements, it also has weight-bearing effects known to slow or reverse bone loss.

Because the exercises are learned slowly, more and more weight is gradually exerted on bones. This gentle form of exercise therapy is ideal for those who have soft bones from the disease, says Suza Francina, Iyengar Yoga Instructor and director of the Ojai Yoga Center in Ojai, California.

Francina uses yoga props such as blankets, bolsters, straps, blocks, and benches to help older yoga students and those who might be weak, stiff, or have injuries or structural imbalances.

Finding a qualified yoga instructor who has a full understanding of osteoporosis might require some work, says Trisha Lamb Feuerstein, director of research for the Yoga Research and Education Center of Lower Lake, California.

Feuerstein encourages potential yoga students to ask an instructor about the depth of her training and watch a class. Training centers and yoga styles known for advanced training standards include Kripalu yoga, Integrative Yoga Therapy centers, Phoenix Rising Yoga therapy, Viniyoga, and Iyengar yoga.

For help locating an instructor or identifying the yoga form best for you, contact the Yoga Research and Education Center at P. O. Box 1386, Lower Lake, CA 95457.

For more information on these and other healers, contact the Office of Alternative Medicine at the National Institutes of Health. Write for their general information package at OAM Clearinghouse, P. O. Box 8218, Silver Spring, MD 20907.

Index

Boldface references indicate illustrations.